Transforming the Doctor's Office

From the parking lot to the exam room, doctors can improve the physical surroundings for their patients, yet often they do not. Given the numerous and varied duties doctors must perform, it may fall to the design profession to implement changes, many based on research, to improve healthcare experiences. From location and layout to furnishings and positive distractions, this book provides evidence-based information about the physical environment to help doctors and those who design medical workspaces improve the experience of healthcare.

Along with its research base, a special aspect of this book is the integration of relevant historical material about the office practice of physicians at the beginning of the twentieth century. Many of their design solutions are viable today. In addition to improving the physical design of healthcare facilities, author Ann Sloan Devlin is the granddaughter, daughter, and niece of physicians, as well as the granddaughter and daughter of nurses. She worked in a hospital during college, and has visited a good many practitioners' offices in medical office buildings and ambulatory care settings. This book addresses an overlooked location of care: the doctor's office suite.

Ann Sloan Devlin is the May Buckley Sadowski '19 Professor of Psychology at Connecticut College, New London, USA. She has published extensively on healthcare environments, investigating how perceptions of the built environment influence judgments of care and comfort. She has written three other books, most recently *What Americans Build and Why: Psychological Perspectives* (2010).

Transforming the Doctor's Office

Principles from Evidence-Based Design

Ann Sloan Devlin

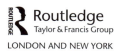

LONDON AND NEW YORK

First published 2015
by Routledge
711 Third Avenue, New York, NY 10017

And by Routledge
2 Park Square, Milton Park, Abingdon, Oxon OX14 4RN

Routledge is an imprint of the Taylor & Francis Group, an informa business

© 2015 Taylor & Francis

The right of Ann Sloan Devlin to be identified as author of this work has been asserted by her in accordance with sections 77 and 78 of the Copyright, Designs and Patents Act 1988.

All rights reserved. No part of this book may be reprinted or reproduced or utilized in any form or by any electronic, mechanical, or other means, now known or hereafter invented, including photocopying and recording, or in any information storage or retrieval system, without permission in writing from the publishers.

Trademark notice: Product or corporate names may be trademarks or registered trademarks, and are used only for identification and explanation without intent to infringe.

Library of Congress Cataloging in Publication Data
Devlin, Ann Sloan, 1948– author.
Transforming the doctor's office : principles from evidence-based design / Ann Sloan Devlin.
pages cm
Includes bibliographical references and index.
1. Medical offices. 2. Medical offices--Design and construction. 3. Evidence-based design. I. Title.
R728.D48 2015
725'.23--dc23
2013038496

British Library Cataloguing in Publication Data
A catalogue record for this book is available from the British Library

ISBN: 978-0-415-84063-7 (hbk)
ISBN: 978-0-415-84064-4 (pbk)
ISBN: 978-1-315-79626-0 (ebk)

Acquisition Editor: Wendy Fuller
Editorial Assistant: Emma Gadsden
Production Editor: Jennifer Birtill

Typeset in Syntax LT Std 10/12 pt
by Fakenham Prepress Solutions, Fakenham, Norfolk NR21 8NN
Printed by Bell & Bain Ltd, Glasgow

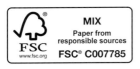

This book is dedicated to the generations of healthcare practitioners in my family.

Contents

Preface	xi
Acknowledgments	xiii

Introduction — 1
    Physicians and their image — 1
    Clues to identity and quality of care — 1
    Changing status of physicians — 2
Role of evidence-based design — 2
The patient-centered care movement, Planetree, and the Center for Health Design — 3
Green design, sustainability, and technology — 5
Americans with Disabilities Act (ADA) and Health Insurance Portability and
    Accountability Act (HIPAA) — 6
The role of evidence — 6
    Causality — 6
    Meta-analyses and multi-method strategies — 8
    Post-occupancy evaluations (POEs) — 9
Unifying themes in this book — 9
    Schemas or mental representations — 10
    Control and competency — 10
    Choice — 10
    Territoriality and personal space — 10
A call to action — 11

1 Office Location, Signage, and Identity: Where and Who You Are — 13
Overview: Schemas and patients' expectations — 13
    The schema: What people expect — 13
    The physician's identity in the early twentieth century — 14
    The physician's identity today — 15
Location — 15
    The implications of location — 15
    Office locations today — 15
    A word about medical malls and their connotation — 16
    Location and wayfinding — 16
    The doctor's office and the cognitive map — 16
Signage — 17
    Signage physicians can and cannot control — 17
    Assessing signage in the vicinity — 17
    Even small places need a signage system — 18
    Types of signs — 19

Your sign location	19
The sign: Historical reflections	23
Signage for group practice	23
Challenges of signage in an office complex	24
Wayfinding schemes in multi-level buildings and complexes	24
Parking	25
Parking, the front entrance, and wayfinding	25
Planning parking and forgiveness	26
Parking: Necessary vs. sufficient	28
Exterior landscaping and image: An overview	28
Outdoor spaces with nature: Importance for patients and practitioners	30
Why nature matters	30
Preferred elements in the landscape	31
The healing garden for outdoor spaces	33
Desirable qualities in outdoor spaces: What people prefer in healing gardens	34
Undesirable qualities in gardens	34
Specific recommendations for outdoor furnishings	34
Wayfinding elements in the landscape	36
Lighting in the garden	38
Further reading	38

2 Arriving, Waiting, and Taking Vitals: Setting the Stage — 39

Overview	39
The spatial continuum: From entrance and reception to interior spaces	40
Arrival	42
Wayfinding: Navigation cues for patients	44
Manifest and latent cues	47
Color as a wayfinding cue: A caution	47
Use of redundant cues	49
The view as a wayfinding cue	50
Reception space: Expectations and functions	50
Reception windows and counters	51
Check-in stations and kiosks	51
Reception area and HIPAA concerns	51
The waiting room: Territoriality, personal space, and privacy	53
Territoriality	54
Personal space	55
Seating and social interaction	56
How many seats do you need?	59
Opportunities for personal control	59
Lighting	62
Personal control	62
Functions	62
Types of lighting	63
Furnishings	63
The Scaffolding functions: Staff preparation and storage areas	64
Vital signs, nursing station, and location	65
Laboratory functions and traffic flow	68

Staff areas	69
Communication: Implications for patient privacy	69
Staff lounge and toilet areas	69
Supply and storage functions	70
The toilet room (restroom)	71
Patients, staff, or both? Public? Private? The restroom locations	73
Patients' restrooms: Private office location vs. public corridor	73
Number of restrooms: Individual occupancy	74
Protocol for leaving the specimen	74
Maintenance, storage, and functionality	74
Lighting	75
Positive distractions and aesthetics	75
Further Reading	75

3 Consultation and Examination Spaces: "You Feel Healthier When You're Dressed"   77

Overview	77
Anxiety and the medical consultation	77
Models of consultation	77
The traditional exam room	78
Exam room layouts	81
"Having a seat at the table"	82
The Jack-and-Jill layout	82
Location of consultation and exam spaces	83
The exam room: Same-handed vs. mirror image	83
Shared functions	84
Functional aspects of the exam room	85
Privacy concerns: Overview	87
Auditory privacy	87
Cell phones and other communication	89
Summary of design considerations	89
The electronic office and doctor-patient communication *(DPC)*	89
Monitor position	90
Illumination: Properties of lighting and dynamic lighting systems	91
Natural light	93
Dynamic lighting	95
Effects of lighting on staff	95
Personalization in the office suite	95
The psychotherapist's office: Continuous consultation and examination	97
The spatial layout	97
The view	97
Design issues in telemedicine and teletherapy	97
Restrooms: Group and individual practice	98
Security considerations: The role of design	98
How furnishings and décor influence clients' judgments of the therapist	99
Consultation and exam spaces: A century ago	99
Who decorates? The silent partner	100
Further reading	102

4 The Ambient Environment: Changing the "Sick People's" Atmosphere	**105**
Overview: The waiting room should "lose its 'sick people's' atmosphere"	105
Ambient characteristics: Control, positive distraction, and personalization	105
Giving patients control and permission	106
The senses: Visual stimulation and positive distraction	106
The 180-degree principle	106
Positive distraction: The debate surrounding television	107
Windows, natural light, and views to nature as positive distractions	110
Access to nature for staff	114
Water as a positive distraction	114
Water: A caution	115
Nature: The real deal	116
The use of plants	116
Substitutes for nature: Art	117
The content of art: Recommendations	118
Too much of a good thing?	118
Visual microaggressions	118
What you display affects patients	119
The displays of early practitioners: Implications for today	119
Self-paced distraction: Reading material	120
Music as positive distraction	120
Preferred types of music	122
Sources of music: The CARE Channel (Continuous Ambient Relaxation Environment)	122
Music: Mode of delivery and sources	122
Exercising control: Having patients bring their own music	123
Complimentary food and beverages	123
Other senses	125
Cleanliness and odor	125
Air quality and odor	125
Aromatherapy	126
Temperature and thermal comfort	126
Cleanliness and carpeting	126
Green cleaning and design	127
Safety in the medical suite: By regulation and by association	128
Safety by design	128
Functionality and safety: Related concerns	129
Closing thoughts	130
Further reading	130
Notes	133
Image Credits	149
Index	151

Preface

In examination rooms, patients' clothing may end up on a chair because the clothing hooks are either inconveniently located or absent altogether. Waiting areas may consist of a series of small alcoves where patients invariably feel cramped; their personal space is restricted. These examples illustrate just a few of the many oversights in practitioners' healthcare offices; from the parking lot to the exam room, doctors can improve the physical surroundings for their patients, yet often they do not. Given the numerous and varied duties doctors must perform, it may fall to the design profession to implement changes, many based on research, to improve patients' healthcare experience and health outcomes. From location and layout to furnishings and positive distractions, this book provides information about the physical environment to help doctors and those who design medical workspaces improve healthcare.

The physical environment is one component of an arsenal to improve not only the quality of the patient experience but also the success and reputation of the physician's practice. Beyond improving patients' immediate experience, attracting and retaining patients matters to hospitals and doctors. With patient satisfaction surveys such as HCAHPS (Hospital Consumer Assessment of Healthcare Providers and Systems) readily available, patients now have standard measures to directly compare hospitals; hospital performance is increasingly transparent. Unfortunately, this ready transparency has not trickled down to evaluations of physicians in their office suites. By offering evidenced-based information, this book enables design and medical practitioners and also patients to assess the environments they create, use, and visit, respectively.

The book's focus is the primary care physician's office practice, whether in a freestanding building or within a hospital complex, but some research related to hospitals more generally is featured. Many of the principles in this book apply to ambulatory care facilities and community health centers as well. Including the hospital-based information provides a more complete picture of what we know from evidence-based design. Some research topics that apply to hospitals (e.g., the role of signage; auditory privacy) also apply to the practitioner's office, community health, and ambulatory care centers. I have also used photographs that come from inpatient settings when I thought the images demonstrated principles that would translate to these smaller venues. This book is timely because medicine is big business, and the role of the physical environment is emerging as an aspect to differentiate providers as well as improve care.

Following the Introduction, each chapter deals with a particular aspect of the patient experience, explains the available evidence in an understandable way, and provides recommendations as appropriate. As an organizational theme, these topics move from public to private space, starting outside with location, parking, landscape, and signage, and moving into the interior spaces in the office suite. A special aspect of this book is the integration of relevant historical material about the office practice of physicians at the beginning of the twentieth century. This material may give practitioners an appreciation that physicians have grappled with similar problems for over a century. Some of the solutions from the past are viable today.

One of the reasons I decided to write this book relates to my family history. Both of my grandfathers were physicians, as were my father and his brother. My mother and her mother were nurses. I worked in a hospital during my college years, and I have lived long enough to visit a good many physicians' offices in medical office buildings and other facilities where primary care is delivered. This book addresses an overlooked location of care: the doctor's office.

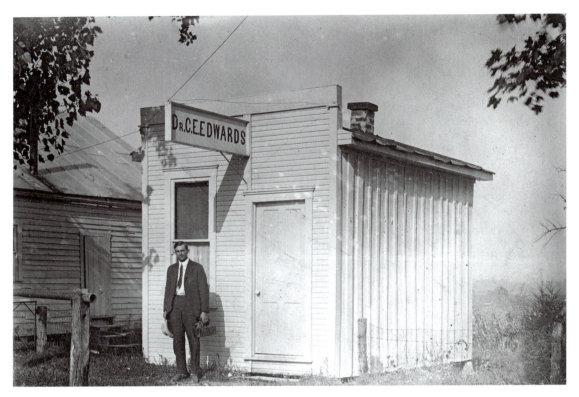

The author's maternal grandfather, Dr Carl E. Edwards, circa WWI.
Location: Central Ohio

Acknowledgments

I want to thank Wendy Fuller, the architecture editor at Routledge, and her senior editorial assistants Emma Gadsden and Laura Williamson, for expertly shepherding this book project to completion. Dennis O'Brien, wayfinder and illustrator extraordinaire, was an important resource for this book. The illustrations he provided and his knowledge of wayfinding programming were pivotal in shaping the content in Chapter 1.

A number of architecture firms provided material and photographs of their healthcare projects. These firms and personnel include those from The S/L/A/M Collaborative (Daniel Fenyn and Tara Calavas); Vision 3 Architects (Keith Davignon); BBH Design (Nicholas Watkins and Trish Coulson); and Interior Architecture & Design, PLLC (IDeA) (Dawn A. Gum). The work of architectural photographers significantly contributed to the quality of this book. In particular I want to thank John Giammatteo, Peter Brown, Aaron Usher, Dawn A. Gum, architects at The S/L/A/M Collaborative, and Nancy Laemle, of Northern Westchester Hospital. Sheila F. Cahnman graciously allowed me to use her exam room layouts. These layouts previously appeared in *Health Facilities Management* magazine, which provided copyright permission. Where no photography credit is given, I was the photographer.

A number of practitioners also allowed me to photograph their offices, including Timothy Barczak, Daniella Duke, Neeraj Kohli, Lloyd McDonald, and Denis Sindel; a number of those images are featured in the book. Mark D'Antonio, Media Relations Coordinator at Yale-New Haven Hospital, accompanied me on a photography tour of the main floor of the facility; Martha Denstedt, Director of Planetree Programs and Services at Griffin Hospital in Derby, Connecticut, kindly arranged a tour of Griffin Hospital for me.

A tour offered at the EDRA 44 conference in Providence, Rhode Island enabled me to photograph the Neonatal Intensive Care Unit of the Women & Infants Hospital of Rhode Island, and the Women & Infants Center for Reproduction and Infertility. A number of those images are used in the book.

Mark Braunstein, who was the Visual Research Librarian at Connecticut College when this book was written, graciously helped to restore the image in the Preface. I also want to thank Connecticut College for a sabbatical in the fall, 2013 semester, when I completed this book.

Finally, thank you to David and Sloan, and to my siblings, who remind me what really matters.

Introduction

> All signs should be neatly made and properly lettered, for even a sign makes an impression, either good or bad, on the public, and first impressions are very enduring.[1]

This comment by the writer of a book entitled *The Physician Himself and What He Should Add to His Scientific Acquirements*, first published in 1882, points to one theme of this book: how something looks makes an impression on those who view it. For that reason we cannot simply ignore the components of impression formation as short-lived. How an office sign looks is not necessarily an indication of practitioners' talent and skill, but in the absence of information about those characteristics, appearance matters. At the beginning of the twentieth century, appearance was extensively covered in advice manuals for physicians setting up practice, such as the manual by Cathell that was quoted to begin this chapter. Unfortunately, such information seems less available today, or at least less effectively put into practice.

Physicians and their image

One hundred years ago, it might have been easier to identify a physician in the community (traveling to see a patient) than today. There was a definite schema of a doctor. Physicians often had a beard and sideburns; even their horse and rig might have been distinctive.[2] The focus in this book is the physical environment, but we should not underestimate the role of the physician's presentation in the success of his practice. In the prevailing wisdom, the physician had about 6–8 years to establish a suitable reputation and practice; if he missed this window, the opportunity to earn a decent living as a physician might have disappeared.[3] The physician's appearance played a role in whether the practice thrived. "Patients are acute observers, and the least thing smacking of vulgarity is repulsive to them."[4]

What was visible outside the practice on the street was important, and practitioners were admonished to avoid a scrawny horse or a tattered carriage stationed in front of the office for any length of time. Again, the astute patient noticed such objects and might assume you had few patients; a physician whose practice was flourishing would know better than to let people think he couldn't afford better.[5]

Clues to identity and quality of care

As these historical descriptions suggest, clues to our personality are transmitted from many aspects of our surroundings and personal appearance; physicians are not exempt from this influence. For example, where the physician's office is located and how it is furnished reflect upon that practitioner and may purposefully (e.g., diplomas) or unintentionally (e.g., magazine subscriptions) communicate aspects of personality. The researcher Samuel Gosling has documented the way in which our surroundings communicate much about us in his popular book *Snoop: What Your Stuff*

Says About You.[6] Attention to the surroundings in which medicine is practiced is an important aspect of a rapidly changing medical landscape. In December 2010, writing for the Whole Building Design Guide of the National Institute of Building Science, Robert Carr[7] commented on cues that signal the quality of care in a facility. These cues start with the signage as you approach the facility, long before you actually enter it. The physical environment does matter, and a significant amount of my research and writing has focused on the role of the physical environment in shaping patients' judgments of the medical facility and the practitioner.

Whether we want to or not, we initially judge a book by its cover or, in this case, healthcare providers by the way their offices look. First impressions count, yet many healthcare providers pay scant attention to the impact of their physical surroundings on patients' impressions of them and their expertise. Physicians and other healthcare providers may need assistance in creating an environment that is welcoming. In other words, they may not know the impact of their offices on judgments people make of them. Among these judgments are the quality of care and the comfort experienced within those office walls. The primary purpose of this book is to help healthcare designers and practitioners create offices that are supportive, welcoming, and functional for patients (and staff), based on the available evidence. This goal is achieved by incorporating research with ramifications for design.

Changing status of physicians

As the practice of medicine changes, so does the nature of the doctor-patient relationship. Paralleling some of the changes in education more generally, the practice of medicine is becoming increasingly consumer oriented. Medicine is a business. We see this consumer culture in the ability of patients (aka healthcare consumers) to compare hospital data on how patients think hospitals perform. We see this in best hospital and best doctor issues in magazines ranging from *US News & World Report* to *New York Magazine*. We are a culture of "best" lists and "Top 10s". We like to be on top and to use the services of those who are rated to be. People shop aspirationally – that is, they shop at places selling goods beyond their financial reach because they can view themselves as members of a more affluent group. Social psychologists explain this behavior using self-congruity theory; we want to see ourselves as more upscale than in truth we are.[8] Why should aspirational shopping be limited to the mall? Medicine is a purchasable service.

Role of evidence-based design

Thankfully, this view of doctors and medicine as unaware of and/or unconcerned with the role of the physical environment is changing. In the last 15–20 years, a movement called evidence-based design has begun to shape research on healthcare environments and change the way hospitals, in particular, are built. Evidence-based design refers to design recommendations produced by research on the relationship between the physical environment and objective outcomes, such as blood pressure or the dosage of analgesics. This evidence-based research shows that healthcare outcomes (e.g., rates of infection) are influenced by environmental design (e.g., the location of sinks in the patients' rooms).

Self-report data are sometimes classified as evidence based and have been used for at least two decades to assess patient experience (e.g., Press Ganey Patient Satisfaction Survey). Such feedback relies on patients' recollections and is just one type of information to consider. Data less susceptible to the factors that distort self-reporting (e.g., social desirability, aka "faking good," or simply forgetting) must be considered. These data are increasingly available through research that associates physiological measures (e.g., blood pressure; heart rate; salivary cortisol levels) with particular design features (e.g., views of nature; single-occupancy rooms). The doctor's skill is certainly the most important but not the only variable that impacts outcomes. There is increasing recognition that the physical environment plays a role as well.

Thus far we know more about differentiation of outcomes between hospitals than between practitioners' offices. One example of evidence-based design related to hospitals is the increase in single room occupancy, its acceptance tied to such recommendations as the 2006 Guidelines for the Design and Construction of Health Care Facilities from the American Institute of Architects. This example supports the argument that, as an increasingly consumer-oriented enterprise, healthcare needs to pay attention to its consumers (its patients); and creating comfortable and non-threatening surroundings is part of its challenge. One way of describing this attention is called patient-centered care. This emphasis on patient-centered care can be translated to the doctor's office suite.

The patient-centered care movement, Planetree, and the Center for Health Design

The Planetree model of patient-centered care emerged in the late 1970s out of the negative hospital experience of a single patient, Angelica Thieriot. Prompted by medical care that in her view lacked humanity, she founded Planetree – a patient-focused approach to the environment of care in which the patient's senses are nourished, rather than depleted. Planetree derives its name from the tree under which Hippocrates taught early medical students in Greece.[9] The Planetree model emphasizes the physical surroundings for both patients and their families. Attention is paid to sights, sounds, and smells. There is artwork in the hallways; music playing softly, often from a grand piano in the lobby; and the scent of freshly baked cookies in the air. Patients and their families have access to an array of amenities, from a medical library and open nursing stations that invite communication about the patient's situation, to the equivalent of room service for meals and a 24-hour visiting policy. There are alternative therapies such as aromatherapy; there are massages; and there are open kitchens where family members can create favorite meals for the patient. Many of these initiatives, including art and music, the medical library, and complimentary beverages and snacks, could easily be incorporated in the physician's office practice. A number of photographs in this book will highlight practitioners' offices with such amenities.

The Planetree model, in many ways, launched the patient-centered care movement and has been adopted by over 100 hospitals or healthcare systems in the United States and over 40 abroad, which are listed on the organization's website. Research has generally indicated subjective improvements in patients' responses to Planetree units, in comparison to non-Planetree units,[10] which is an important outcome, but there is also more convincing evidence that hospital stays are reduced when the Planetree model is adopted.[11]

When cost reductions were not sufficient for hospitals to balance their budgets (post-1997 and the Balanced Budget Amendment, with concomitant reductions in Medicare reimbursement), hospitals sought ways to increase revenue. This idea of attracting patients by improving all aspects of services struck a chord, particularly with the growth of healthcare consumerism. Hospitals have been compared to brands, and building a brand identity – one that may feature the kinds of services that the Planetree model offers – is one successful approach.[12]

Another contribution to research on patient-focused care comes from the Center for Health Design, established in 1993 as a nonprofit organization with the specific goal of using design to improve healthcare outcomes. One of the Center's important contributions is the Pebble Project (from the idea that a single pebble thrown on the water will generate ripples). In this case, the pebble is research. Like ripples on a pond, a single research project has grown into many. The purpose of this research includes improving patient outcomes but also retaining staff (which can be linked to the physical surroundings in which care is delivered), attracting more patients (the bottom line is important), improving efficiency, and increasing productivity. The Center for Health Design website features the "Ripple Database," a searchable database being developed for research on evidence-based design. This database is an important resource for practitioners and designers.

One example of the kind of research undertaken by the Pebble Project involves Bronson Methodist Hospital, in Kalamazoo, Michigan. When Bronson built a new facility with single room occupancy for patients, it recorded an 11 percent drop in infection rates over the old hospital,

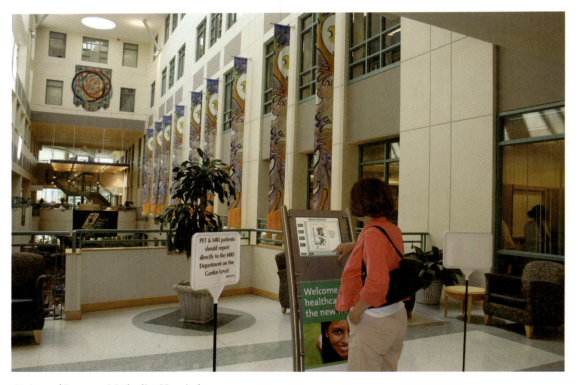

Atrium of Bronson Methodist Hospital.
Location: Kalamazoo, Michigan.

which had semiprivate rooms. Admittedly the construction costs were higher with single room occupancy, but the expenses were to be recouped through a variety of improvements, including fewer medication errors, shorter hospital stays, and fewer patient transfers, among others.[13] If you walked into the lobby of this hospital, with its emphasis on patient and family-centered care, you might think you had landed in a first-rate hotel.

There is a large atrium, bright colors, and extensive interior landscaping; music is often being played at a grand piano. There is also a first-rate cafeteria that draws people from the community. Healthcare facilities, from large hospitals to small doctors' offices, have the potential to be welcoming, and such environmental support ought to be possible on the scale of a doctor's office. Other initiatives that emphasize the role of the physical environment to varying degrees are the Idealized Design of Clinical Office Practices (IDCOP), sponsored by the Institute for Healthcare Improvement,[14] and six quality aims for care from the Institute of Medicine (IOM), part of the National Academy of Sciences. An article titled "The Role of the Physical Environment in Crossing the Quality Chasm," was able to show how the six IOM quality aims could be translated into physical design, for example through standardization of room design and single room occupancy.[15] These examples of national initiatives show that the role of environmental design is being recognized.

Green design, sustainability, and technology

Other recent developments with the potential to impact smaller-scale facilities involve green design and sustainability. The focus of the Hospital for a Healthy Environment (H2E) program, renamed Practice Greenhealth in 2008, is to reduce toxic waste in healthcare settings, including totally eliminating mercury waste, coupled with disseminating education and prevention information.[16] Examples of sustainability efforts usually target large institutions and can be innovative. The new Fort Belvoir Community Hospital south of Washington, DC, a facility for active and retired service members and their families, features sustainability innovations like an upturned curved roof that captures rainwater. This rainwater in turn feeds into an irrigation system that nourishes a healing garden where patients can sit; the healing garden can also be seen from all waiting areas.[17] The lessons from Practice Greenhealth could be incorporated on a smaller scale in primary practice facilities. Green design and sustainability will increasingly trickle down to smaller facilities, whether through selecting windows to reduce energy consumption, planting shade trees near the office, or using biodegradable paper products.

Technology may influence sustainability; it also dramatically affects everyday life in the form of access to the Internet. Patients are increasingly savvy in their use of the Internet to research their symptoms, which creates new challenges for practitioners. For the first half of 2009, more than 50 percent of Americans aged 18–64 used the Internet to look up health information.[18] For Medicare-eligible professionals in private practice, as elsewhere in medicine, electronic medical records (EMRs) are mandated by the Affordable Care Act in order to avoid financial reductions. Beyond EMRs, an example of incorporating technology would be a dermatologist photographing a suspicious lesion and uploading that digital image to the patient's electronic file in real time in the exam room. That photograph is then available for comparison on subsequent visits. Practitioners must plan for technology, both how it will be used and where it will go (e.g., needing a server room). There are also policy decisions to be considered – for example whether practitioners want the waiting room to have computers available to patients as well as Wi-Fi accessibility throughout the office.

Americans with Disabilities Act (ADA) and Health Insurance Portability and Accountability Act (HIPAA)

Practitioners may be well aware of the Americans with Disabilities Act (ADA) requirements that impact the design of their office, from exterior issues like the accessibility of ramps needed to enter the office to interior issues like the handicapped-accessible dimensions of bathrooms. Even the Health Insurance Portability and Accountability Act (HIPAA) has an impact on the physical environment of the office. For example, are computer screens with patient records visible to those checking in at the reception desk? In one dental practice, the reception area had just been renovated with a new configuration that placed a bank of computer screens directly across from the patient check-in window. When this potential breach in patient confidentiality was pointed out, the partners in the practice had the receptionist's windows frosted and etched to shield the computer screens from those checking in. Sometimes the cure is worse than the illness; now patients feel the need to duck down beneath the frosted glass to make initial contact with the receptionist.

The role of evidence

Increasingly, practitioners will need to stay abreast of the research literature. Given the amount of time it takes to become an expert, which some researchers estimate at ten years culminating in the accumulation of 50,000 facts, it is unlikely that architects or healthcare providers will have the time (or inclination) to master the nuances of research design and statistics. As an alternative, it is possible to grasp the fundamental concepts that guide research and the evaluation of its quality with a modest time commitment. Topics important to understand include basic research design (and related issues of correlation and causation), meta-analysis, significance levels, and the design-oriented strategy of post-occupancy evaluation. Designers and healthcare providers desiring more in-depth understanding of these issues should consult introductory texts in research methods. Journal articles are also appearing that help architects and designers better understand how to evaluate the quality of published research.[19]

Causality

At the heart of understanding research is the degree to which one can attribute causality to the variables under investigation. When the research design involves a true experiment, where conditions are manipulated and participants are randomly assigned to those conditions, there might be a reasonable degree of certainty that the manipulated variable caused a particular outcome. A variable that is manipulated is called the independent variable; the outcome measure – that is, the behavior or measure that is assessed, such as number of falls or patient satisfaction – is called the dependent variable (its value "depends" on the manipulated variable).

Often, when an experiment is conducted, the researcher selects a between-subjects experimental design. What this means is that the participants are randomly assigned to the conditions (two or more). Using patients as our participants, one group could be assigned to condition 1 (semiprivate rooms); other participants to condition 2 (private rooms); and still other participants to condition 3 (open units). In this example, our independent variable is the room occupancy (number of people sharing a room). Ideally in this scenario, patients would have the same diagnosis and be as similar as possible in all background characteristics. Potential outcome measures might be the number of days patients took to recover, the number of falls patients experienced, or the degree of patients' compliance judged by nursing staff. When research of this type is conducted, the statistics used report the means and standard deviations of the dependent variables for each condition. Usually some form of analysis of variance is used, ranging from *t*-tests to the multivariate level; such analyses test for significant differences between means in sets of data.

When variables are not manipulated and people are not randomly assigned to particular conditions, you have correlational research. In correlational research we can only be sure about the association or relationship between variables; we cannot claim that one variable caused a change in another because we have no manipulation. There are no independent and dependent variables. For example, one might assess the degree of relationship between patients' satisfaction with their doctor visit (indicated on a survey) and the distance people had to drive to get to the office (which patients could report). You might find a significant inverse relationship between satisfaction and the number of miles driven (i.e., the more miles driven, the lower the degree of satisfaction). A correlational statistic that measures the degree of relationship between two variables is called for in this situation. The most commonly reported correlational statistic is the Pearson product-moment correlation, also called Pearson's *r*. People also might ask the question whether one variable (such as miles driven) predicted an outcome variable (such as satisfaction). In this case, the statistical approach is regression. In correlation and regression nothing is manipulated, and the statistic used reports the relationship over all participants, not in terms of groups. No causality can be inferred.

A challenging concept to understand is that even when statistical analyses are used that treat people as members of a group, unless those people were randomly assigned to that condition and an independent variable was manipulated, causality cannot be claimed. In our example, we could take people who drive to the doctor's office and put them into two groups: people who drive ten or fewer miles to the office and people who drive more than ten miles. We could do an analysis asking if those two groups differ in their level of satisfaction with their office visit experience. We would report the satisfaction for each group in terms of means and standard deviations. Can we claim a causal relationship between group membership (over or under ten miles) and satisfaction? No, we cannot, because these people were not randomly assigned to where they live and hence the number of miles they had to drive to the office. When designers read the empirical literature and want to understand the degree to which a particular design feature caused or impacted a particular healthcare outcome or behavior, careful attention must be paid to the research design that was employed. The message to remember is: design implications for data that lack manipulated variables are limited; some other variable that has not been assessed could explain the relationship of interest.

A significant challenge in evaluating the impact of design on healthcare and/or attitudinal outcomes is the healthcare setting itself. It is difficult to conduct experiments in healthcare settings. A new facility could be constructed and outcomes for that facility assessed (e.g., number of falls, number of infections, degree of patient satisfaction). In such situations so many variables remain unmeasured that we cannot claim causality; we cannot attribute outcomes solely to specific design features in these cases. Moreover, when facilities are renovated, it is hardly ever the case that only one variable is changed, making it impossible to isolate the causal variable in the design.

Meta-analyses and multi-method strategies

What strategies are available to address some of these research challenges in healthcare settings? There are a number of ways, two of which will be briefly highlighted. One is meta-analysis; the other is multi-method research. Meta-analysis is sometimes called the study of studies. In meta-analysis no new data are collected; instead the researcher is looking for an estimate of the relationship between variables, based on a large number of previously published studies. To calculate the size of this relationship, called the effect size, the researcher searches through the literature (using databases such as PsycInfo, Scopus, and PubMed) looking for studies on a particular topic, such as the relationship between room occupancy and level of nosocomial or hospital-acquired infection (HAI). In this search the investigator is compiling information about the number of participants involved in each study, the research strategy used (for example if and how participants were assigned to rooms), the mean of the infection rates in the experimental group (e.g., patients in single-occupancy rooms) and the mean of the infection rates in the control group (e.g., patients in larger-occupancy rooms). An effect size is computed for each study; then the effect size for all of the studies together is computed. The strength of meta-analysis is that it takes into account all of the empirical research on a given topic. Further, the arithmetic calculation takes into account the size of the sample in each study, weighting it accordingly. When the overall effect size is calculated, the result gives you a much better sense of the strength of the relationship between variables (e.g., room occupancy and HAI) than you would have from a single study. In other words, you can have more confidence in the results of a meta-analysis than from an individual study. For that reason, conclusions based on meta-analyses deserve our attention.

A second way to deal with the challenges inherent in research on healthcare settings is to look for research using multiple approaches, hoping that the data will converge (point toward the same conclusion). For example, in a multi-method approach, there might be subjective data collected, where patients and staff fill out a survey indicating their level of satisfaction with a particular design feature, like the location of a restroom adjacent to the waiting room vs. adjacent to the exam rooms in a practitioner's office. There might also be more objective data collected, such as the number of times staff must provide directions to the restroom. In addition, there might be multiple sites where data were collected. In other words, the more ways and times you can measure the impact of the design issue, the more confidence you typically can have in the outcome.

Whatever your research strategy, the statistical test will typically report what is known as a *p* value, or a probability value, of a result meeting a specific criterion or cutoff, usually set at .05 or less. This .05 value, in essence, states that there are only 5 chances in 100 (.05) that the result of interest occurred by chance. In other words, whether for a correlation (a measure of relationship) or for a measure of group difference, when the statistical analysis shows that the numerical result has achieved or improved upon this .05 requirement, you refer to results as being "significant."

Note, statistical significance and practical significance are not equivalent. In the example of correlation we used earlier, imagine your analysis showed a significant relationship [r (200) = −.30, p = .04] between satisfaction with the office visit and number of miles driven to get there. In this example, 200 is the number of participants (patients), −.30 is the Pearson's *r* value (the degree of relationship), and *p* = .04 is the significance level achieved (which has met the criterion of .05 and is even *less* likely to have occurred by chance than that, at only 4 chances in 100). However, r^2 (called *r*-squared) is the amount of variability in the relationship that is explained by knowing the relationship between satisfaction and number of miles driven. Here, r^2 = −.30 x −.30, or .09. Not very impressive. What .09 shows is that only 9 percent of the variability in people's satisfaction with their office visit can be explained by knowing the number of miles driven. Many other factors may have influenced their level of satisfaction, from the time they had to wait to see the practitioner to the prognosis delivered in the visit. In reading the literature, therefore, it is important to keep track of the *p* values and of the *r* values; a finding can be statistically significant but have little explanatory power. In other words, a statistically significant finding, especially from a correlational study, does not necessarily translate into powerful design guidelines.

Post-occupancy evaluations (POEs)

Of the research traditions in the field of architecture, POEs probably have the greatest familiarity. POEs typically involve assessing a variety of outcomes after a building or space is occupied. Doing this research costs money; often a client is unwilling to pay for such research. As a result, fewer of these evaluations are conducted and published in the literature than designers would like. As important as these studies are, it should be noted that POEs are plagued by the kind of correlational problems we addressed earlier. In the language of research design, a POE often reports a case study; it is typically research about a single facility and may report behavior only following construction or change. There are ways in which POEs can yield more valid data (i.e., in which the data actually measure what we claim they do). More valid data are yielded when the research approach includes measurements over time, for example. One such approach is known as a pre-post design [measure before (Time 1) and after (Time 2) change]. Nonetheless, without a control group (in this case a similar facility that is subject to measurement before and after but does not include renovation), we cannot truly be convinced about the impact of specific design changes on behavior. Fortunately, as the climate about conducting research in healthcare settings becomes more favorable, POEs are being conducted that involve more multi-method approaches and come closer to what might be described as true experiments.

Conducting good research is difficult, and the healthcare setting presents incredible challenges for research because of the difficulty in manipulating variables and randomly assigning people to conditions in the context of delivering care. Nevertheless, as healthcare practitioners and administrators become more persuaded by the need to understand how the built environment affects a whole range of outcomes, some of the obstacles to doing good research should disappear. Understanding the basics of research design and attributions of causality, the issue of significance, and the kinds of studies (such as meta-analysis) that improve the validity of the results can lead designers to be more confident about the conclusions of published research.

Unifying themes in this book

In this book, a series of themes related to human needs are highlighted to unify design goals across different topics. These themes are: the schema or mental representation needed to understand the environment, an evolutionary product of having limited processing capacity; the human need to exert control in the environment (related to competency motivation); the need to have choice in a physical setting; and the need to establish territoriality and manage personal space.

Schemas or mental representations

In their books *Humanscape: Environments for People* and *Cognition and Environment: Functioning in an Uncertain World*,[20] Stephen and Rachel Kaplan help us understand how humans evolved in a dangerous and uncertain world, in the process developing into creatures that were model makers. As model makers, acting efficiently and yet at the same time accurately guaranteed survival. In this description of survival the schema, or the mental representation of the environment, is central to understanding how humans operate. The schema is an important concept when applied to design. Based on their experiences, people form representations of the world (e.g., where restrooms are likely to be located in a public facility) and have expectancies about how an environment will probably look (e.g., waiting rooms of physicians typically have chairs lining the walls). Understanding the powerful role of the schema can help designers anticipate what people expect and use that knowledge to create understandable environments.

Control and competency

The human need to exert control in the environment is also a fundamental tendency. Following Freud, psychoanalytic theory developed a more optimistic view of human nature through the work of Robert White, who discussed the idea of competency motivation or the need to have an effect on the world.[21] Humans derive pleasure from mastery, figuring out how things work, finding their way, and a host of other interactions with the environment. Healthcare environments are among the most deficient, likely second only to correctional facilities, in terms of providing opportunities for mastery. Keeping in mind this need to demonstrate mastery and to be effective can help designers think about ways in which to help people succeed, whether it is finding the location of an office or figuring out where to leave a specimen in the toilet room (i.e., restroom).

Choice

Related to the idea of competency is the idea of choice. People enjoy choosing among alternatives (up to a point); this activity gives them a sense of control over the environment and is another aspect of mastery. In choosing whether to adjust the illumination on a table lamp in the waiting room, the fact that we have the option to do so is almost as important as whether we actually make that change. This idea comes from the psychologist Martin Seligman who, with Steven Maier, developed the theory of learned helplessness.[22] This theory explains that over time, when people repeatedly cannot influence the outcome of events, they stop trying. They have learned to be helpless. The schema of the healthcare environment activates a feeling of such helplessness, but designers can provide opportunities to act on the environment.

Territoriality and personal space

Two final concepts important in design of the physical environment are territoriality and personal space, which also relate to control. Humans are hierarchical animals with status issues figuring prominently in who we are and who controls space. Humans want to occupy and control space, in the process giving access to some and not to others. Altman[23] identified three different kinds of

Introduction

territories: primary, secondary, and tertiary. A space that an individual almost exclusively controls, such as a bedroom, is a primary territory. When an individual frequently controls a space, such as a chair in a classroom where that person almost always sits, it may be described as a secondary territory. Others may use that space (sit in the chair if they arrive first), but there is an unspoken agreement that the space is reserved for the usual occupant. In tertiary territories, such as the waiting rooms of healthcare facilities, every person has an equal right of access and choice. Being cognizant of humans' territorial nature will help designers maximize patients' territorial rights by providing sufficient choice in the more public spaces of the office.

Personal space – which Altman also discussed, following the work of Robert Sommer[24] – is about having a transportable invisible boundary around the self and is one factor that determines how comfortable we are when people approach us. Generally, only others with whom we are intimate may enter our invisible spatial bubble. In the context of the healthcare environment, that personal space boundary may be encroached upon if there is not enough seating in the waiting room. There are other times in healthcare settings when we may have to relinquish control of that personal space altogether. This kind of shift in boundaries happens during a physical exam because the physician performing the exam has a special role vis-à-vis our health. Nevertheless, anxiety often accompanies such violations of personal space. Aspects of the examination room can lessen this anxiety through positive distractions such as views to or pictures of nature. Sufficient seating and an organization of seating that values territoriality and personal space in the waiting room can also lessen anxiety. Keeping in mind these principles, from the schema as a mental representation of our expectations to the spatial realities of personal space, can help the designer create offices that match human needs.

A call to action

This book is a call to action for designers and the healthcare providers they serve. It is time to consider how the physical surroundings of the office suite affect the experience of patients, staff, and even physicians themselves. Physicians may be surprised that they, too, are affected by the surroundings in which they practice medicine. This book is a guide to designing physical settings that reduce patients' anxiety, elevate staff morale, and signal that physicians care about patients.

Using research, the book addresses how the physician's office is experienced, from the role of signage in locating and identifying the facility to the sense of welcome in the doctor's consultation space or personal office. The focus is specifically on the office practices of primary care physicians, whether in a freestanding building or a complex. Research done in hospitals is included because the majority of evidenced-based recommendations come from these larger facilities. These outcomes may translate into recommendations for smaller-scale facilities (e.g., the role of signage; views to nature). A special aspect of this book is the integration of relevant historical material about the office practice of physicians at the beginning of the twentieth century. In my judgment, not only does this material make the book more interesting to read, but it also provides an understanding of how physicians have grappled with the same kinds of problems for over a century.

Chapter 1 focuses on issues of location (where the office is located), associated issues of exterior signage, parking, landscaping, and exterior spaces, such as gardens.

Chapter 2 deals with the entrance and reception area, waiting room, staff preparation and storage area, and toilet room; it includes a discussion of the traffic flow through the office, interior spatial configuration (how these spaces are connected), and related signage. Ambient features are touched upon here but are fully presented in Chapter 4.

Chapter 3 focuses on the consultation spaces in the office, including the exam room and the doctor's personal office. Issues of visual and acoustical privacy are addressed, as is lighting. The chapter includes a special section on the psychotherapist's office because the use of the office for therapy creates special demands on space, décor, and privacy issues related to traffic flow.

Chapter 4 addresses the role of the ambient environment including artwork and other positive distractions such as music. Views to nature; odor and cleanliness; thermal comfort; green issues; and safety are also covered.

Each chapter includes recommended readings on the topics covered in the chapter.

Office Location, Signage, and Identity: 1
Where and Who You Are

Overview: Schemas and patients' expectations

"If it is not obvious where to park, if there is no room to park when you get there, if you stumble into the back door looking for the front entrance, or if the entrance is badly lighted, your guests have been subjected to a series of annoyances which will linger long in their subconscious."[1] In this quotation the distinguished landscape architect Thomas Church was writing about arriving at a residence, but his admonitions apply to the practitioner's office.

Like guests' expectations upon arrival, this chapter focuses on patients' expectations about where doctors' offices are likely to be located, the meanings ascribed to such locations, and the role of signage in helping patients reach these destinations. In addition, it covers aspects of external landscaping and parking. Providing an historical perspective, the chapter also includes examples of how and where physicians established medical practice at the beginning of the twentieth century. The emphasis here is on primary practice physicians with offices located in a small complex of medical buildings, a freestanding building, or within the hospital itself. The focus is on the physical context where care is delivered and how physicians are consequently perceived.

The schema: What people expect

Based on their experience, people expect physicians to look a certain way (e.g., to wear a white coat) and proceed a certain way (e.g., to first ask about symptoms). When we go out to dinner in a restaurant, there is a predictable chain of events that psychologists call a script or an event schema. Similarly, an office visit to a doctor involves a particular sequence of activities: check in with the receptionist, wait for a length of time in the waiting room, and have your vital signs taken; speak to your physician about the reason for your visit; pay in some form; and exit the way you entered. We have a script for our visit. Not only do we have expectations about the activities, but also about the appearance of the office and its surroundings.

A major theme in this book is the role of schemas, or mental representations of knowledge, that people have about their world and how these schemas shape our reactions to physical environments and those who inhabit them. Humans are limited information processors; we cannot process all of the stimulation around us at a given moment in time. One of the major reasons telephone numbers and zip codes are short is our inability to remember much more than seven digits, written about by the psychologist George Miller.[2] With auditory (e.g., conversation) and visual (e.g., signage) interference in the environment, that limit is likely to be even lower.[3] Further, despite what those born toward the end of the twentieth century (the Millennials) think, multitasking is not making us more efficient or able to perform diverse tasks at the same time.[4] Thus, layout and signage must compensate for our memory limitations.

Fortunately we function in a reasonably predictable although complex world, at least with regard to the built environment. We know that hospitals are not typically located in quiet residential neighborhoods, given traffic and ambulance noise. The predictability of our world is advantageous because humans are quite easily overcome by information. To manage the complexities of our environment, we rely on schemas or representations of both how things usually are and where things usually are. The human brain has modules to register these categories of information, known respectively as the "what" and "where" systems.[5]

The physician's identity in the early twentieth century

The practice of medicine was significantly less complex 100 years ago than today. When my maternal and paternal grandfathers practiced medicine in Brownsville, Ohio and Clarksburg, West Virginia, respectively, beginning in the early 1900s, practice was either in a physician's home or a small office (see Preface illustration); many practitioners were not yet licensed. My paternal grandfather's major means of transportation was a horse, later replaced by a bicycle because it was more convenient than waking the attendant in the barn to saddle the horse for night calls.[6] Eventually my grandfather acquired an automobile. When he retired in 1952, medicine had been transformed from those early years.

A century ago, there were perhaps three or four times more doctors than were needed,[7] competition for patients was strong,[8] and as a rule, physicians were advised not to send patients elsewhere for fear income would be lost. The concern about how to make a living was reflected in the titles of books written to help the physician, including Cathell's 1882 *The Physician Himself and What He Should Add to His Scientific Acquirements*, Wood's 1903 *Dollars to Doctors or Diplomacy and Prosperity in Medical Practice*, Mathews' 1905 *How to Succeed in the Practice of Medicine*, and journals such as Albright's *Office Practitioner*. Today, as then, there is concern about how to make a living, especially in this era of managed care.

Where physicians practice has also changed since my grandfathers' era. Today physicians' offices are typically in medical office buildings or connected to the hospital. Sometimes they are in renovated houses but certainly not in the physician's home unless the practice is psychotherapy; even then, home offices are the exception.

Despite these changes, many of the tasks in setting up practice in a private office remain much the same as 100 years ago; doctors must select the location of the office and furnish it. Coursework on how to establish an office is not a formal academic subject, and the environment reflects this neglect. How these offices look, both from the street and as you enter, often disappoint us, if we judge by what patients say. In research on waiting rooms,[9] one of the participants commented that the decorations looked like torture devices. We can change that; some of the early twentieth century recommendations provide advice that makes sense today.

The medical office in the home was the common practice before the turn of the twentieth century, yet few patients visited doctors in their office; if you were "sick enough to have the doctor," you essentially couldn't get out of bed. Doctors came to your house. When the office was outside the home it was typically located on the second floor of a building, above a commercial enterprise such as a bank or store.[10]

The physician's identity today

Who the individual is as a practitioner is reflected in all aspects of his or her behavior and surroundings. The location, the look of the office building's exterior, and the interior of the office itself all reflect on the physician. The architecture of the building, the landscaping, and even the lighting communicate aspects of identity. All aspects of medical practice comprise a system of identity.[11]

Location

The implications of location

For city practice in the early twentieth century, the recommended location for the office was near a major thoroughfare, but not directly on it, and in the central part of town. Such a location was convenient for both the physician and his patients; being near but not on a major thoroughfare provided greater privacy. A convenient and central location was important because the patient might remember that location, but perhaps not your name.[12] Other advice comes from Cathell in 1882: "If you were to locate on a back or unfrequented street, or other out-of-the-way place, it would naturally suggest to the public either defective ambition or distrust of your own acquirements."[13]

The office should be in a place that communicates safety as well as convenience; that is, located in a place where it is safe to get out of the car, taxi, bus, or subway, and safe to walk on the surrounding streets. This recommendation seems obvious, but competing interests such as real estate costs (the cost/square foot) and/or availability of parking may override factors reflecting patients' concerns and perspectives.

Being a patient is stressful. Designers and healthcare practitioners can and should take steps to reduce that stress. Helping people to more easily find the physician's office is one area amenable to stress reduction. Yes, by the second visit, the location is not a mystery; but the first visit is important in beginning a positive relationship. As one author commented, "Signs are a form of public relations."[14] When efforts are taken to create a clear signage system and tactful messages, users may sense the physician cares about them and understands how important it is to reduce stress.[15] Related to this idea of public relations is the recognition that people don't like to feel inadequate or incompetent; they like to figure out how things work. Having to ask for directions may make people feel insecure and increase stress.[16] This idea reflects the human need to exhibit mastery, a theme presented in the Introduction that can help guide design decisions.

Office locations today

There are two major kinds of locations for physicians today. One choice is a location near (or in) the hospital where they primarily practice; the second is centered in the community from which they expect to draw most of their patients. In either location, wayfinding (the process of finding your way from an origin to a destination) may be a challenge. For that reason, aspects of wayfinding (e.g., considerations of location and signage) are covered in this book. Even in a relatively small community hospital, wayfinding issues may be complex because hospitals are typically multi-part structures. Some of the factors that operate to make wayfinding difficult in large facilities also operate in small facilities. These factors include terminology as well as renovations and additions that often complicate the layout.[17]

A word about medical malls and their connotation

We began this chapter talking about schemas, and there is some concern that the commercialization of medicine as represented in the medical mall (doctors with offices located in commercial malls) may tarnish the relationship between the patient and doctor. Such malls do have assets – for example, their recognizability (i.e., the mall is a familiar building type), parking, and prominent signage. On the other hand, the potential instability of leases and the issue of the surrounding context may weaken the credibility of the medical profession. A given mall may not house nail salons, tattoo parlors, or pawn shops, but a preponderance of retail venues may create a commercial schema that unfavorably envelops the physician. In the book *Medicine Moves to the Mall*, medical malls are described as "docs-in-a box": "In a perverse irony, America's most prestigious profession utilized one of the culture's least exalted built forms to reorder its relationship with its clientele."[18] Physicians need to carefully consider the larger context of their offices. There are implications not only for the connotation of the surroundings, but also for the wayfinding or navigation difficulties the locations present, discussed next.

Location and wayfinding

Years ago, the urban planner Kevin Lynch[19] talked about the anxiety that surrounds getting lost and the structure of the urban form that helps us understand urban environments and form mental maps (our schemas or internal representations, also called cognitive maps). If we are able to form a coherent mental model of the environment, our ability to find our way will be supported. Lynch's focus was the larger urban environment and the streets, districts, and landmarks that structure our experience. Graphic designers have also emphasized the role of signage in its ability to evoke a sense of order and calm as people are guided through a facility where signage serves a variety of functions, from welcoming and identifying to warning.[20]

The doctor's office and the cognitive map

How does this issue of the ease with which cognitive maps are formed relate to the doctor's office? The doctor's office is part of a larger environment – it is on a street (or accessed from a street), in a neighborhood, located in part of a community (town, city), and likely accessed by an Interstate. Some people might consider the idea of finding your way to be trivial in this era of GPS navigation systems, mounted in your car or available as an app on your smartphone. Programs provide many features – for example, position tracking in real time and directions, which can be either text or voice guided.

Not all patients have access to such systems, and these systems do not always function. Even when people consult Internet features like MapQuest or get directions from Google, the maps typically do not provide the level of detail of an office complex or building interior. The option to "view map" on a practitioner's website may not even work.

If they have websites for their office practice, 1) physicians should make sure that they offer functioning downloadable maps to direct patients once they reach the site itself. If the office is located within a medical office campus, 2) physicians should provide downloadable maps of the campus that indicate a) which building it is and b) which suite it is within that building. If space is rented in a medical complex, whether a large building or a series of buildings, 3) it is important to work with the owner of the building(s) to address some of these larger legibility issues. It is in the owner's and the physician's interest to reduce the wayfinding challenges for patients, and graphic and/or web designers can be contracted for these maps. For all of these reasons, it is important to consider the wayfinding challenges presented by the physician's office location in the absence of technical support.

Signage

Signage physicians can and cannot control

Before focusing on signage installed on their site, physicians and designers need to look farther afield at the signs they cannot control. Taking inventory of these uncontrollables will give physicians a better sense of where their own signs should be placed and how their own signs should look to establish their own signage program. Yes, signage program. Signage is not simply a matter of installing one sign near the road to identify the destination (the office location). A signage program takes into account the number and placement of exterior and interior signs and includes a consideration of what wayfinding information staff provide and how. This chapter highlights those exterior signage issues.

Assessing signage in the vicinity

Physicians should make note of the posted signage in the area within a half mile of their office. That signage includes everything from road signs to the signs identifying chain stores, restaurants, and even gas stations. Questions to ask include: 1) What other signs may compete with the physician's sign(s)? 2) Would these competing signs block the physician's sign(s)? 3) Are the colors similar?

When there are many pieces of information in the environment (think back to the limitation of about seven digits), visual clutter makes picking out the physician's sign a challenge. In this situation, physicians might consider installing a larger sign or more signs than originally planned. One caution is in order; physicians should not succumb to what is known as the "Las Vegas syndrome," which occurs with over-signing (i.e., posting too many signs).[21]

Signage matters. Looking at what else has been used in the community and beyond helps to give a sense of the level of taste in a community (range of size, colors, and materials). Communities have character; they have levels of taste reflected in their architecture. Tastes within a geographical region and urban-rural differences may also dictate the kind of material used to construct the sign (e.g., wood vs. brick vs. metal), such as this metal sign from downtown Vancouver in contrast to one from a small town in the Northeast (see Figure 1.01, top and bottom images, respectively).

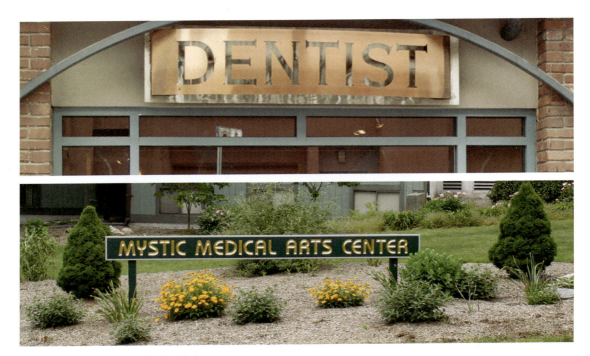

Figure 1.01: *Examples of regional signage.*
Location: Vancouver, British Columbia (top); Mystic, Connecticut (bottom).

Even small places need a signage system

Common refrains such as "everyone knows where we are because we've been here for years," "after patients arrive it will be obvious where we're located in the facility," or "signage systems are just for really large facilities" are sometimes used to avoid wayfinding issues.[22] The information provided in a signage system must yield ONE destination. Even a small place (a single building for a solo practitioner) needs a signage system to help patients reach this destination. Tasks for the initial visit include: 1) finding the office, 2) determining where to park, 3) locating the entrance (if you have parked in back, there may be more than one entrance), and 4) ascertaining where to check in. What kinds of aids assist patients in these tasks? Even figuring out where to park may be difficult in a setting where public and private parking spaces coexist. The factors that influence decisions about this wayfinding system start before the curb when physicians consider the surrounding neighborhood and the challenges for wayfinding it may create. A sign is not simply an incidental. A sign makes a claim to identity with its placement, size, and typeface; such an identity becomes even more important with the proliferation of mergers and acquisitions of hospital systems and the growth of specialized ambulatory treatment centers, such as the cancer care center seen in Figure 1.02.

Signage systems must be updated from: 1) personnel changes, 2) weather-related wear, or even 3) destruction. One practitioner became tired of replacing his office sign, located near the road, after inebriated drivers speeding on weekend nights routinely knocked it down. Without a sign, the office is hard to find.

Office Location, Signage, and Identity   19

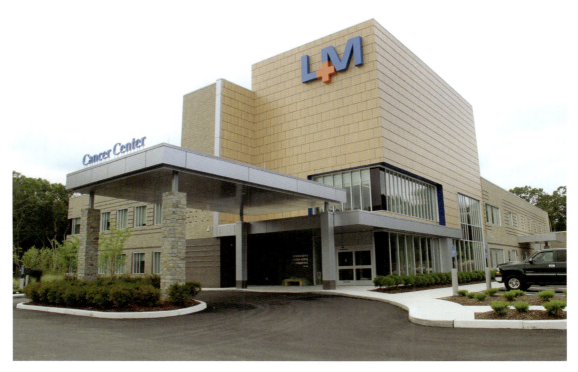

Figure 1.02: *Logo illustrates strong visual identity.*
Location: L&M Cancer Center, Waterford, Connecticut.

Types of signs

Most authors who devote books to signage divide signs into categories based on function for example: 1) identification, 2) direction, 3) warning, and 4) regulation, including those where specific actions are prohibited (e.g., Staff Only). Others list identification, direction, prohibition, information, and status.[23] Figure 1.03 shows another common functional scheme (identification, direction, description, and regulation). Some authors reduce wayfinding signs to just two categories: direction and identification.

An important principle is that signs for direction must be visually distinctive from signs that identify destination.[24] A second principle, which is ubiquitous in the literature on wayfinding, is that signage must be presented at choice points.[25] Whenever a decision needs to be made about turning or continuing ahead, a directional sign is required. With its white arrows, Image 2 in Figure 1.03 shows what is to be found continuing ahead and what is to be found by turning right.

Your sign location

The sign identifying the physician's office falls into the category of identification. The sign may be constructed according to known standards and recommendations about the size, spacing, and color contrast of letters; some of these variables are dictated by municipal codes. For readability,

Office Location, Signage, and Identity

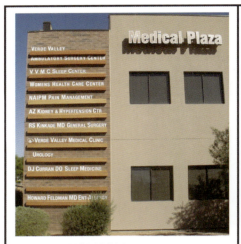

1. IDENTIFICATION:
   Naming Locations: Names, Addresses
   Designating Areas: Parking Levels; Rooms

Verde Valley Medical Plaza, AZ

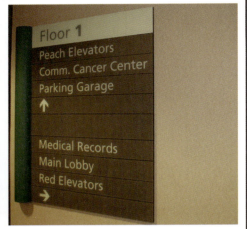

2. DIRECTIONAL: Pointing to Destinations

Lawrence & Memorial Hospital, New London, CT

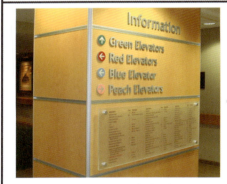

3. DESCRIPTION: Detailed Information: Maps, Directories, Hours

Lawrence & Memorial Hospital, New London, CT. The bottom half is a Directory.

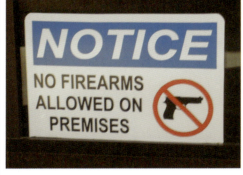

4. REGULATION:
   Commands, Prohibitions, Warnings

Manzanitas Medical Plaza, AZ

Figure 1.03: *Signage categories.*
Plate credit: Dennis O'Brien, Maps and Wayfinding, LLC

the sign should be close to the road/street (municipal codes will dictate how close), paying particular attention to obstacles that might impede viewing. In other words, the distance from the sign to the curb is not the only consideration.

This book emphasizes best practices, but it is occasionally useful to show the other end of the spectrum and the negative impact that follows. In Figure 1.04, the sign identifying an office park

Office Location, Signage, and Identity 21

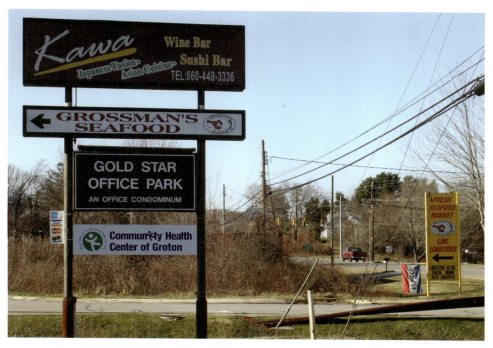

Figure 1.04: *Signage clutter.*
Location: Groton, Connecticut.

(housing many medical practices) has to compete with three other signs (four, including the fresh seafood market sign). This example shows the challenges of being "seen" against a backdrop of visual clutter.

To address these issues, some commonly endorsed principles for exterior signs are:

- To locate signs perpendicular to the direction of movement and sight (so people can see the sign without turning their heads).

- To the extent the physician can control the signage, he/she should provide advance directional signs to help people get ready to turn, especially when the turn is around a bend and could surprise a driver who is not prepared.

- To consider the distance the driver (viewer) would have, the angles from which the sign would be viewed, and any obstructions that might be present (e.g., overhanging trees) in sign placement near the road/street.

- To consider lighting the sign at night[26] (as was the practice in the early twentieth century) (see Figure 1.05 for effective approaches). The lighted sign in the top photo illustrates a number of good design practices: good figure-ground contrast, size (large enough to be seen from the street), and simplicity. The bottom image shows how welcoming a facility can be when it is lighted at night, especially when evening appointments are offered and/or the community uses the facility for meetings, as is the case in the Thundermist Health Center, shown here.

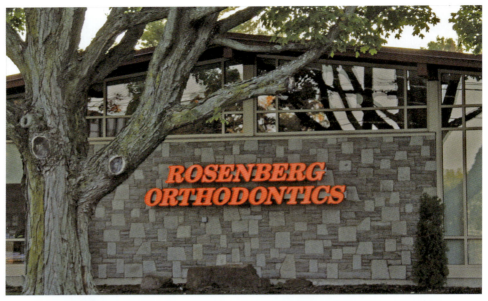

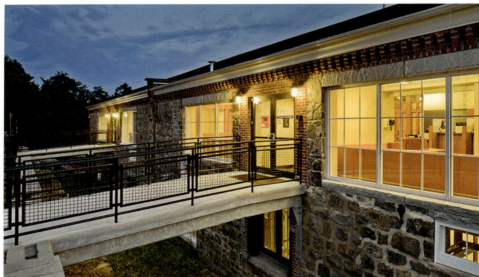

Figure 1.05: *Advantages of lighted signs.*
Location: West Hartford, Connecticut (top); Thundermist Health Center, West Warwick, Rhode Island (bottom).
Architect (bottom): Vision 3 Architects.
Photo credit (bottom): Aaron Usher III Photography

Signs have a visual personality (see, for example, Figures 1.01 and 1.02); the physician needs to acknowledge the cultural context within which he/she practices (at the very least the physician should know what that context is before rejecting or endorsing it). Size is also related to cultural preferences; historically, Americans have adopted a bigger (and more) is better philosophy, which

Office Location, Signage, and Identity

often extends to signage. Constraining the "more is always better" mentality is important. A reasonable suggestion is to follow what is known as the KISS principle (Keep It Simple Stupid). People underestimate the importance of leaving space on a sign, for example.[27]

The sign: Historical reflections

In the early 1900s, the office sign garnered a great deal of the physician's consideration. Mathews commented that you were not done with your office until you had considered "the *sign*" (its importance indicated in italics), a decision of great importance to the practitioner starting practice.[28] Cathell recommended two signs: for daytime, an exterior sign with a black background and gold letters posted on the street-facing facade of the building; for night, a sign of glass with black letters visible in the window. To be visible at night, the office needed to be lighted. "Have your office lighted punctually every evening at the proper hour, and in all other respects let it show attention and system."[29]

Signage for group practice

Today, if you are in solo practice, a common approach to identity is to simply put your name and possibly your specialty on the sign:

>   Herbert Sloan, MD

>   Practice Limited to Thoracic Surgery

But what if the physician is part of a group practice with two or more members, a more likely possibility given the declining number of solo practitioners? Listing each practitioner may overload the sign. In that situation, having a group practice name or building complex identification makes good sense from a wayfinding standpoint, as two quite different signs indicate. In Figure 1.06, there is already competition on the sign from other services; in the bottom image of Figure 1.01, the distance from the road would make individual practitioner names virtually unreadable. In these instances, group practice names make more sense. In addition, when personnel change (practitioners come and go), the group practice name still functions.

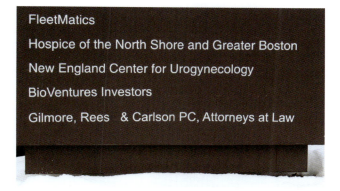

Figure 1.06: *Sign illustrates competition and the role of a group practice name. Location: Wellesley, Massachusetts.*

Challenges of signage in an office complex

Wayfinding is often more complicated for a practice in an office complex than in a single building. When buildings have multiple tenants, the need for a strong visual identity may increase. In these more complex situations, the basic principles are the same, but they have to be considered at each level. At each choice point, the practitioner should ask: What information on this sign gives the patient the information he or she needs to reach ME without false steps? If an office is located in a complex, practitioners with a website can direct patients there to download a map. Lacking a website, practitioners can mail or e-mail patients a map with the layout of the buildings to facilitate wayfinding. In addition to the obvious benefits for patients, providing such helpful information also says something important about physicians: they care about their patients.

Wayfinding schemes in multi-level buildings and complexes

In a single building with multiple floors, using a numbering scheme with a maximum of three digits (e.g., Suite 391) is the limitation recommended by some graphic designers.[30] When you have multiple buildings, or buildings with multiple parts, the recommendation is to use symbolic systems that typically reflect an ordered basis (such as A, B, C; 1, 2, 3; South Pavilion, North Pavilion). The signage system in Figure 1.07 incorporates repeated wayfinding elements: the use of color (green) for the South Pavilion; the shape of the sign itself, which has a curved top, and the white lettering.

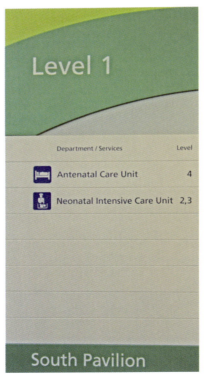

Figure 1.07: *A signage system with repeated elements.*
Location: Women & Infants Hospital of Rhode Island, Providence, Rhode Island.

Office Location, Signage, and Identity

As the sole wayfinding cue, color is not recommended for such signage systems. In the previous example (Figure 1.07), it is important to note that the color would never appear without the label "South Pavilion." Most designers caution against color used alone because 1) there are no universal associations to color, 2) those who are colorblind would have difficulties, and 3) there are age-related changes in the ability to detect colors. At the same time, as we have seen, color can be used in conjunction with alphanumeric systems. In image 3 of Figure 1.03, the color green is used as part of the wayfinding scheme, but it appears in conjunction with the word "elevators" – as is true of all of the other colors (red, blue, peach). When introducing a new wayfinding system in a medical campus or multi-part building, a pilot project (which could be as simple as putting up paper versions of the elements of the plan) is recommended. It is easy for wayfinding systems in multi-part buildings to go awry.

Symbol systems that use pictograms, (i.e., pictures that represent or symbolize a function) are fairly common, such as the universally understood sign for a women's restroom. When such symbols become inventive, trouble follows. Often such symbols are not understandable without accompanying text. Many symbol systems are destined to fail because their meanings are ambiguous, conflicting, too abstracted, or even have poor figure-ground contrast.[31]

Parking

Parking, the front entrance, and wayfinding

Signage needs to indicate where the building is on the site and where the parking is located. These signs are considered major directional signs and are often at the edge of the property and visible when entering the site (where adjacent streets connect to the property). Secondary aspects of parking indicate locations of the handicapped spots; they can also indicate traffic directions so that those entering the site prepare for whatever actions are required (e.g., turning).[32]

Talking about the characteristics that make Planetree facilities welcoming, Arneill and Frasca-Beaulieu note that the parking and lobby experiences are the first impressions the patient receives: "Immediate, well-marked parking, combined with a covered drop-off, helps ensure a positive impression and minimizes frustration."[33] Essentially, in their view, you strive for an experience similar to that approaching a nice hotel or spa that emphasizes service; they also recommend that the entry be scaled to humans (see Figure 1.08). The use of a porte cochère in Figure 1.08 also protects patients from the elements, whether sun, rain, or snow, depending on the climate.

Signage consists both of explicit labels and implicit expectations, a major point in this chapter in our discussion of schemas. What are the characteristics of a main entrance? We might answer that it is a focal point, often with double doors, perhaps with porte cochère or overhang (the implicit message), with a label that states "Entrance," "Main Entrance," or sometimes "Enter here" (the explicit message). Other expectations include that an entrance is likely the first turn available off the approach road; the passenger drop-off is facilitated if the traffic pattern is counterclockwise.[34]

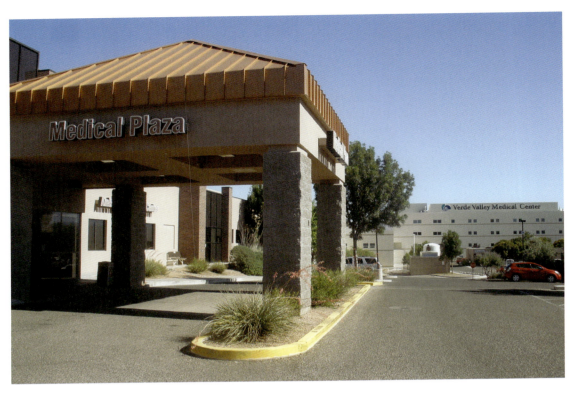

Figure 1.08: *Illustrates welcoming porte cochère.*
Location: Verde Valley Medical Plaza, Cottonwood, Arizona.
Photo credit: Dennis O'Brien, Maps and Wayfinding, LLC

Planning parking and forgiveness

When planning parking, one aspect to consider is the ability to correct a mistake; if people turn in the wrong place, what are their options? Must they exit the site and re-enter? Can they circle around back and try again or must they back up and turn around? Can people reverse direction? Are there warnings in advance if such actions are not possible? In other words, how much forgiveness is there in the parking plan?

A recommendation from Kevin Lynch, the late urban planner, is to cluster groupings of cars in six to ten spaces per grouping to avoid a sense of being overwhelmed.[35] Doing so may also help to manage scale by managing the density of cars, which may in turn limit the number of people you have to encounter in a given area of the parking lot. When the scale is managed in this way, people may have more sense of control. Figure 1.09 from Griffin Hospital, a Planetree affiliate facility in Derby, Connecticut, nicely illustrates this kind of grouping. In addition, seating and trash receptacles are provided and, not apparent in the photographs, there is music. A number of small speakers dispersed throughout the parking lot broadcast the same easy listening music from a cable provider that is used in the facility itself. As you pass the speakers, the music becomes audible.

Office Location, Signage, and Identity 27

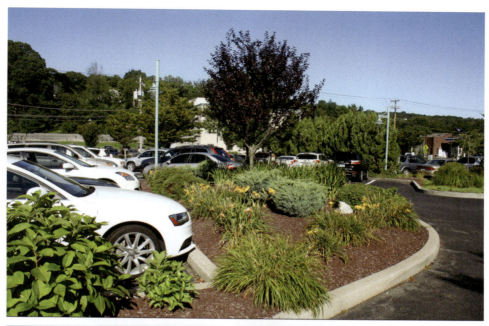

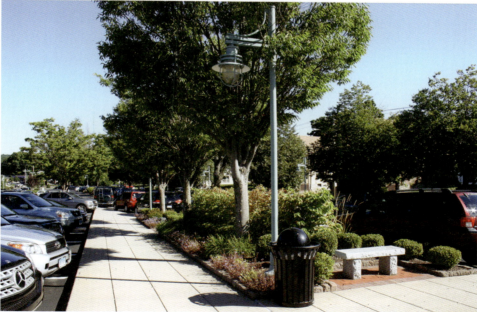

Figure 1.09: *Clustered parking manages people and information. Location: Griffin Hospital, Derby, Connecticut.*

Parking: Necessary vs. sufficient

There is a difference between the number of parking spaces that meet the zoning regulations and what is sufficient for patients. The parking lot dimensions and number of spaces may meet zoning requirements, but the arrangement may still create a tight fit for patients both in turning into and backing out of parking spaces. Older patients who do not qualify for handicapped stickers may still have mobility challenges related to the turning radius the parking lot requires.

Consideration of what is called universal design – which refers to design that is accessible to every person, independent of physical, mental, or other challenges – is appropriate in parking. The philosophy speaks to designing environments and products for everyone, whatever one's age, ability, or individual circumstances.[36]

In addition to considering the turning radius in the parking area, another safety consideration is the relationship of the parking to the main entrance. Handicapped accessible spots will be located near the main entrance (just visible on the right in the example provided by Figure 1.02); other patients may park in front or back lots and need to walk to the entrance.

- How safe is the walk from these lots to the entrance? Would cars driving to and from these parking lots pass by pedestrians?
- Are sidewalks provided for people to walk from the parking areas to the entrance?
- If there is a sidewalk, can it accommodate those with mobility supports (i.e., walkers, wheelchairs) or even two such users passing each other on the same sidewalk?
- Is there covered outdoor seating for people who might wait at the entrance for their ride home or for public transportation?

Related to this, entrances designed for those with accessibility challenges should not look second-rate in comparison to entrances for those without challenges, even when ramps have been added to older structures to comply with ADA requirements. In Figure 1.10, although the rise over run (i.e., pitch) prevented an installation at the front of the building, the incorporation of plantings along the edge of the ramp reinforces the attention given to users with mobility challenges.

Exterior landscaping and image: An overview

The upkeep, pruning, and extent of landscaping all play a role in our judgment of the practitioner. Landscaping also plays a role in enhancing the visibility of the office building. Plantings can direct the eye of the patient to the main entrance; in particular walkways and shrubbery can be used to guide the patient to the front door, as in Figure 1.11.

Landscaping factors vary in terms of how easy they are to control. Even when aspects (such as topography) cannot easily be controlled, other aspects can be used in a compensatory fashion. For example, when the office building is located on an elevation lower than the entrance, this difference creates a less positive image. Carefully maintained trees and plantings can compensate for the elevation.

Office Location, Signage, and Identity 29

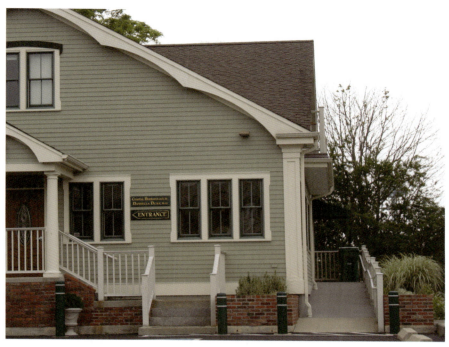

Figure 1.10: *Attention to ramp entrance through plantings enhances patient-centeredness. Location: Coastal Dermatology, Mystic, Connecticut.*

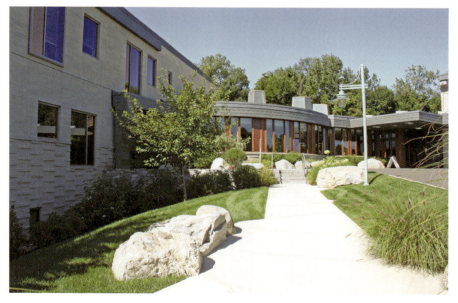

Figure 1.11: *Using plants and walkways to direct patients. Location: The Center for Cancer Care at Griffin Hospital, Derby Connecticut. Architects: The S/L/A/M Collaborative.*

Some aspects of landscaping may enhance the practitioner's image, even if they are controlled by others. If the office is located next to a nature preserve or undeveloped wooded acreage, for example, this context reflects favorably on the physician's practice, as seen in Figure 1.12. This office is located next to wetlands and provides what one might consider a borrowed view. This view is not only visible for patients in the waiting room, as seen in Figure 1.12, but the staff work area provides an even more expansive view of the water.

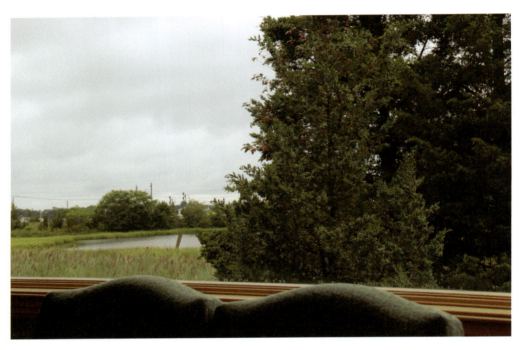

Figure 1.12: *A "borrowed" view visible from the waiting room.*
Location: Coastal Dermatology, Mystic, Connecticut.

Outdoor spaces with nature: Importance for patients and practitioners

Over the last two decades, recognition of the positive role that nature plays in human well-being, and specifically in healthcare settings, has grown.[37] That recognition notwithstanding, a challenge faces the solo or small group practitioner who wants to provide outdoor spaces for patients, visitors, and staff to use and enjoy either on their way to an appointment, waiting for a ride home, or during the course of a break, in the case of staff. In the battle between parking and usable outdoor space, parking often has priority. The usability of outdoor space is often an afterthought. The waiting room is not the first cue about practitioners' attitudes toward their patients; outdoor spaces designed for use by patients and staff speak to the caring nature of the practitioner.

Why nature matters

The research of Stephen and Rachel Kaplan on the benefits of nature[38] focuses primarily on cognitive outcomes, such as attention restoration which involves restoring our ability to focus

Office Location, Signage, and Identity

our attention in a directed manner after it has been depleted. One could argue that attention restoration would be valuable in reducing the kind of stress experienced in healthcare settings. Other research, including Ulrich's seminal study[39] of a view out of a hospital window, shows that exposure to nature has the capacity to improve healthcare outcomes – for example, the level of analgesics requested during recovery. From this domain of research, the message for providers and designers is to carefully consider the role of nature in the site.

Preferred elements in the landscape

In the research of the Kaplans and others in the same vein, studies consistently point to a preference for water in a scene. Another preferred aspect is having a degree of openness (the vista) in the setting. People like nature that is well tended (not weedy),[40] and they like water that looks clean.[41] People seem to like vegetation to match the season in which it is viewed (e.g., blooming flowers in the spring and early summer). Thus, the seasonality of the office landscape and whether it is planted to show seasonal change[42] is relevant. If possible, practitioners should incorporate water elements (e.g., fountains; small fish ponds) and select plants that peak during different seasons. Figure 1.13 illustrates a wonderful combination of blooming flowers and a water element outside an office building in downtown Vancouver.

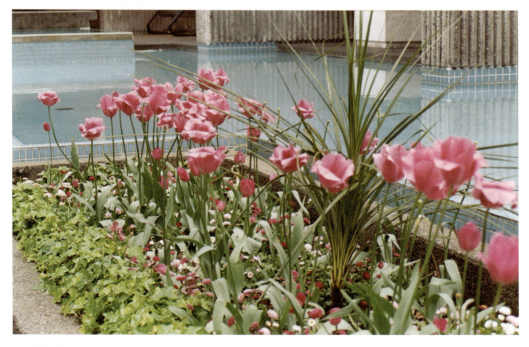

Figure 1.13: *The power of nature through color and water. Location: Downtown Vancouver, British Columbia.*

The two images in Figure 1.14 show the same healthcare facility in different seasons, demonstrating the capacity of water to provide restoration throughout the year.

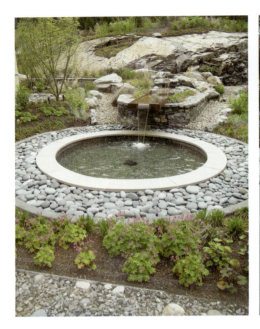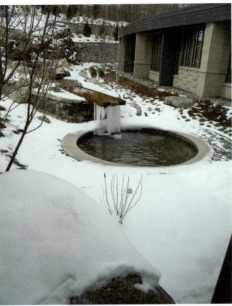

Figure 1.14: *Nature can be restorative year-round.*
Location: The Center for Cancer Care at Griffin Hospital, Derby, Connecticut.
Architects: The S/L/A/M Collaborative.
Photo credit (left and right): The S/L/A/M Collaborative

Not all landscape elements need be large or dramatic to be effective. A small water element could provide visual restoration (see the images in Figure 1.15), as could a water element as part of an outdoor seating area. The example in Figure 1.16 from Vancouver comes from the Dr. Peter Centre for people living with HIV/AIDS.

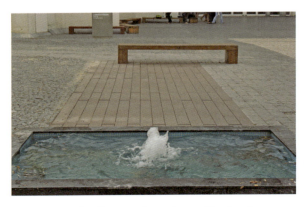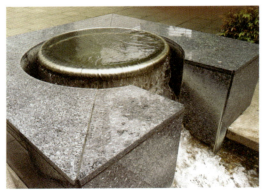

Figure 1.15: *Small water elements provide visual engagement.*
Location: Lisbon University Institute, Lisbon, Portugal (left); urban plaza, Seattle, Washington (right).

Office Location, Signage, and Identity   33

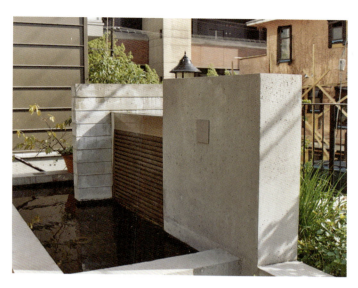

Figure 1.16: *Soothing water element in an outdoor seating area. Location: Dr. Peter Centre, Vancouver, British Columbia.*

The healing garden for outdoor spaces

The concept of a healing garden is most closely associated with the work of Clare Cooper Marcus who, with Marni Barnes, published a seminal work entitled *Healing Gardens: Therapeutic Benefits and Design Recommendations* in 1999.[43] Practitioners may think of healing gardens and gardens more generally as places appropriate for large facilities, but Cooper Marcus and Barnes define a garden as "any green outdoor space within a healthcare setting that is designed for use."[44]

In my view, any garden has the potential to become a healing garden; placing gardens within the context of modern healthcare settings emphasizes their potential to heal. In the view of Cooper Marcus and Barnes, gardens provide stress reduction and are designed for staff as well as patients. A series of studies by Cooper Marcus and her colleagues point to the same conclusion: respondents describe settings with nature as a location for stress reduction.[45] The authors say such outdoor spaces can be used for passive (e.g., sitting) or quasi-passive (e.g., strolling) activities. Importantly, such spaces should be visible from inside the facility; a number of studies point to underuse of garden spaces when people are unaware the spaces exist.[46]

When a garden is designed to meet human needs in terms of choice (e.g., of seating and activities), privacy (e.g., screening and enclosure), and positive distractions (e.g., vistas, fragrant plants, a range of colors), one could argue that it has the potential to be restorative. Ulrich takes that view as well. In presenting his theory of supportive gardens and their effect on health outcomes, Ulrich makes points that overlap with many of the themes in this book. To the extent possible, Ulrich says these spaces should foster: 1) "Sense of control and access to privacy"; 2) "Social support"; 3) "Physical movement and exercise"; and 4) "Access to nature and other positive distractions."[47] In the context of the doctor's office, the sense of control, access to privacy, access to nature, and other positive distractions may be appropriate targets for design efforts.

Desirable qualities in outdoor spaces: What people prefer in healing gardens

Tying in our principles, choice should be provided in the outdoor garden spaces. This recommendation encompasses all kinds of choices: choices of seating, choices of view, and choices of microclimate. Research by Cooper Marcus and Barnes[48] indicates that the garden qualities most often mentioned as being positive are the elements of nature (trees and plants) and features engaging the senses (auditory, olfactory, tactile). Patients should see flowers and their colors, greenery, birds, and squirrels. Patients should feel fresh air, being warmed by the sun or cooled in the shade. Detecting the fragrance of flowering trees and plants is desirable as well.

Undesirable qualities in gardens

The qualities to avoid, Ulrich[49] says, are negative distractions in gardens, and he includes in this list urban noise, smoking, and the potential for sunlight to have an adverse impact. Again, choice is a key variable in avoiding negative outcomes. Shade as well as light must be provided. Sculpture can also be viewed as a negative distraction, especially if its meaning is ambiguous and might be interpreted negatively. As Ulrich notes, it is likely that if someone has to ask what the sculpture depicts, it may not be appropriate in a healthcare setting. People tend to apply their current mood in ambiguous situations when cognitive resources are depleted. If you are depressed, a piece of art that is ambiguous may elicit negative emotions, matching your current mood state. Cooper Marcus and Barnes also comment that whatever symbolic meanings are communicated in the garden setting, they must be "unambiguously positive."[50] In a related point, the authors emphasize the use of the familiar, for example local materials, as reassuring.[51]

Guidelines[52] from Cooper Marcus and Barnes help designers enhance outdoor spaces for patients and visitors. Planning for such usable outdoor spaces has to be a goal from the very beginning of the project. Further, living in particular climates provides challenges to make the outdoor space welcoming and usable 12 months of the year. More shade might be required in the southwest; in the northeast, less screening might be needed and the sun might be more desirable. Different microclimates can be created within the setting. They caution that changes in grade should be carefully evaluated in terms of presenting challenges of accessibility. Other recommendations are handrails along paths and walkways wide enough to accommodate two wheelchairs, which means at least five feet. Guidelines by Carpman, Grant, and Simmons include many of the same ideas.[53] Respondents in research conducted by Carpman *et al.* preferred a great deal of vegetation (trees and shrubs) around private seating areas.

Specific recommendations for outdoor furnishings

Benches and tables are recommended by Cooper Marcus and Barnes, as are wind shelters and gazebos that can protect users from harsh conditions. Both of these aspects are seen in Figure 1.17.

To add coherence to the setting, consideration should also be given to the site vocabulary, including trash receptacles and light fixtures. Trash receptacles should be provided within the garden areas as well as by the front entrance.[54] The very creative and aesthetically pleasing trash enclosure in Figure 1.18 (from Lisbon University Institute, in Lisbon, Portugal) demonstrates that even this aspect of healthcare facilities need not be unsightly if approached with ingenuity and perhaps a bit of whimsy.

Office Location, Signage, and Identity 35

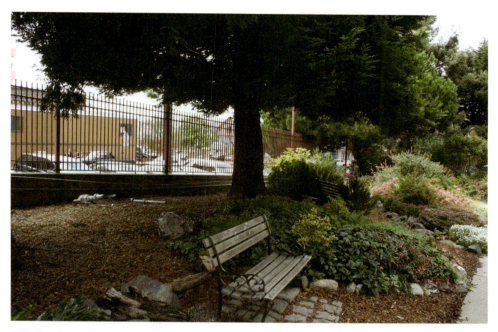

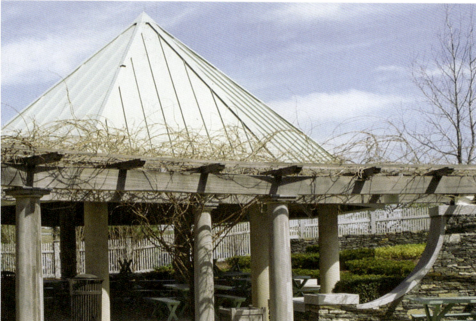

Figure 1.17: *Varieties of outdoor seating elements.*
Location: Comfort Garden, San Francisco General Hospital, San Francisco, California (top); Hasbro Children's Hospital, Providence, Rhode Island (bottom).

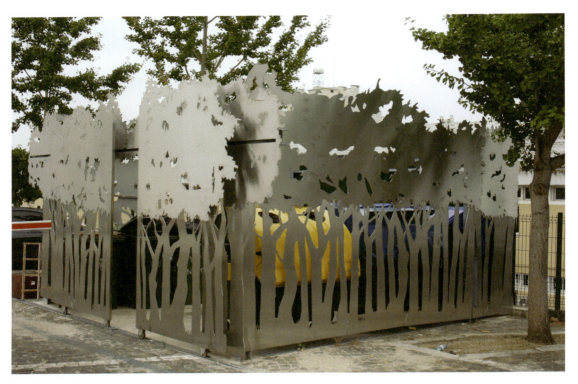

Figure 1.18: *Whimsical and attractive trash enclosure. Location: Lisbon University Institute, Lisbon, Portugal.*

In addition, designers and practitioners might consider having a toolshed (and mulch) near the location of a large on-site industrial trash bin. Consideration could be given to recycling containers and containers for the proper disposal of medical waste that complies with the Occupational Safety & Health Administration (OSHA) and local, state, and federal regulations, although such disposal is typically contracted out.

Carpman *et al.* provide a useful list of characteristics of furnishings for outdoor spaces in healthcare settings, and one of the major themes that emerges is choice. There should be choice in the location of seating – some along circulation paths to facilitate people watching but some in private areas for time spent more contemplatively; and choices of seating group sizes, from seating for just one to two people up to seating for larger groups of five to six people. Their research showed that in a range of furniture choices, the clear winner was a curved slatted wood seat with wood arms.[55]

Wayfinding elements in the landscape

In the context of outpatient care for a solo practitioner or small group practice, the idea of having outdoor spaces intended for patient and visitor use may be unfamiliar. Providing places to sit and paths that lead there are the most obvious clues to intended use. With regard to wayfinding,

Office Location, Signage, and Identity   37

Cooper Marcus and Barnes state that "focal elements for orientation, such as a central feature, marked entry treatment, clear path system, and set boundaries, help to reduce confusion and anxiety."[56] Even fencing could be used to reinforce the visual landscape and the facility's identity, as seen in Figure 1.19 from the Hasbro Children's Hospital in Rhode Island (top image) and Yale-New Haven Hospital (bottom image).

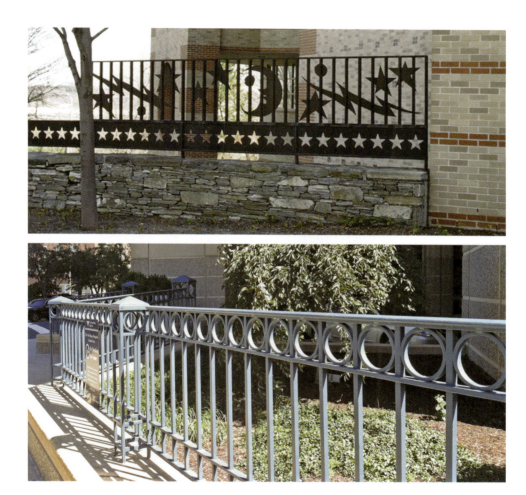

Figure 1.19: *Fences provide thematic coherence and assist wayfinding.*
Location: Hasbro Children's Hospital, Providence, Rhode Island (top); Yale-New Haven Hospital, New Haven, Connecticut (bottom).

Consider how views to nature can promote wayfinding by opening up a vista. In planning the landscape to support wayfinding, designers need to consider the views that are being created and where they lead the patient. Paths from the parking lot should lead the patient to the front entrance without the need for explicit signage (refer to Figure 1.11).

Lighting in the garden

It is unlikely that the garden space would be used at night. Still, lighting should be provided along the paths that lead from the building entrance to the parking area. During dark and stormy days and with the end of daylight saving time, these areas may be dark when the last patient leaves the office, and sufficient lighting most certainly would be an issue for staff.

Further Reading

American Hospital Association. *Signs and Graphics for Health Care Facilities*. Chicago: American Hospital Publishing, Inc., 1979.

Berger, Craig. *Wayfinding: Designing and Implementing Graphic Navigational Systems*. Hove, UK: RotoVision SA, 2005.

Calori, Chris. *Signage and Wayfinding Design: A Complete Guide to Creating Environmental Graphic Design Systems*. Hoboken, NJ: John Wiley & Sons, Inc., 2007.

Carpman, Janet Reizenstein, Myron A. Grant, and Deborah A. Simmons. *Design that Cares: Planning Health Facilities for Patients and Visitors*. Chicago: American Hospital Publishing, Inc., 1986.

Cooper, Randy. *Wayfinding for Health Care: Best Practices for Today's Facilities.* Chicago: Health Forum, Inc., 2010.

Cooper Marcus, Clare, and Marni Barnes. *Gardens in Health Care Facilities: Uses, Therapeutic Benefits, and Design Considerations*. Martinez, CA: Center for Health Design, 1995.

Cooper Marcus, Clare, and Marni Barnes (Eds). *Healing Gardens: Therapeutic Benefits and Design Recommendations.* New York: Wiley, 1999.

Follis, John, and Dave Hammer. *Architectural Signing and Graphics*. New York: Whitney Library of Design, 1979.

Gesler, Wilbert M. *Healing Places.* NY: Lowman & Littlefield Publishers, Inc., 2003.

Harkness, Sarah P., and James N. Groom, Jr. *Building without Barriers for the Disabled*. New York: Whitney Library of Design, 1976.

Lidwell, William, Kritina Holden, and Jill Butler. *Universal Principles of Design*. Gloucester, MA: Rockport Publishers, Inc., 2003.

Meuser, Philipp, and Daniela Pogade. *Construction and Design Manual: Wayfinding and Signage.* Berlin: DOM Publishers, 2010.

Mollerup, Per. *Wayshowing: A Guide to Environmental Signage Principles & Practices.* Baden, Switzerland: Lars Müller Publishers, 2005.

Pollet, Dorothy, and Peter C. Haskell (Eds). *Sign Systems for Libraries: Solving the Wayfinding Problem.* New York: R. R. Bowker, 1979.

Smitshuijzen, Edo. *Signage Design Manual*. Baden, Switzerland: Lars Müller Publishers, 2007.

Trulove, James Grayson, Connie Sprague, and Steel Colony. *This Way: Signage Design for Public Spaces.* Gloucester, MA: Rockport Publishers, 2000.

Uebele, Andreas. *Signage Systems & Information Graphics: A Professional Sourcebook.* New York: Thames & Hudson, 2007.

Arriving, Waiting, and Taking Vitals:
Setting the Stage

Overview

Even for the "routine" annual physical, patients worry. Reducing this anxiety is not a trivial concern; patients are sometimes so anxious they cannot process the medical information they hear.[1] When anxious patients miss vital information, healthcare outcomes can be affected. This chapter will examine how practitioners and designers can lower patients' anxiety by focusing on the environment, including its layout and the opportunities for personal control, as the patient moves through the office. Areas encountered by patients, including the reception desk and waiting room, nursing/vital signs station, and the restroom, are covered. Areas for staff – nursing preparation and supply as well as lounges – are included. Ambient features of the environment, including positive distractions such as art, are mentioned but discussed in detail in Chapter 4.

Office visits will likely take longer in the next few years, given the shortage of doctors[2] that is predicted; patients are likely to wait not only for an appointment but also once they arrive on site, which will add to their anxiety. Increasingly, evaluation is creeping into every aspect of medicine; evaluation pressures underscore the importance of reducing patients' anxiety and increasing patients' satisfaction to provide the most effective climate for treatment and the most positive feedback for physicians. The qualities of the offices described here can improve physiological indicators such as heart rate as well as psychological indicators such as mood.[3] Practitioners are likely to be rated more positively in the process.

Consider a patient saying, "I need to know how much you care before I care how much you know," attributed to the leadership expert and pastor, John C. Maxwell. One measure of care is attention to the physical surroundings of patients. It may be hard for physicians to appreciate that the office environment reflects upon the skill of the physician, at least in patients' minds. The physical environment communicates organizational values; physicians need only look to their own communities to be convinced that hospital administrators see this connection. Significant amounts of money are being spent on the public and private spaces in hospitals, from lobby areas that look like ski lodges with flagstone fireplaces (see Figure 2.01) to single patient rooms with views to nature, plasma TVs, and on-demand restaurant-like menus.

In an article suggesting that doctors, like it or not, are judged like books – by their cover – the author describes her negative reactions to an orthopedist's small waiting room where her son went for evaluation, with "gray walls, dull carpet, seven or eight straight-backed chairs lining the walls and a small portable television on a table next to the reception window blaring a Food Network cooking show."[4] Consequently, the author and her son sought another opinion.

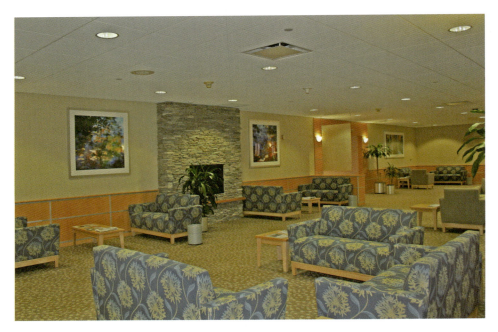

Figure 2.01: *Lobby welcomes patients, families, and visitors using residential materials and furnishings. Location: L&M Hospital, New London, Connecticut.*

This mother's reflection is anecdotal, but empirical research also underscores the relationship between satisfaction with the physical environment and outcomes. Across seven outpatient practices, researchers from Cornell looked at the relationships between physical attractiveness and waiting times, and the outcome of perceived quality of care for patients.[5] In this study, 75 percent of the patients' time was spent waiting; patients spent about one-third of that time in the exam room by themselves. The rated attractiveness of the physical environment was positively related to a reduction in patient anxiety and the overall patient-quality index. Similarly, in research on the waiting rooms of 35 practitioners, respondents judged these waiting rooms and found that aspects, such as attractive lighting, colorful furnishings, neatness, and displayed artwork, were associated with the quality of comfort and care expected. Respondents reacted negatively to those waiting rooms characterized as dark and sparse (e.g., with wood paneling) and those that looked strange and uncomfortable (e.g., with swords displayed on the wall).[6] Why might the physical environment matter so much? Patients can directly perceive how their surroundings look; in contrast, the technical aspects of their visit, such as terminology and procedures, may be much less understandable. Patients therefore rely on what is accessible to them.[7]

The spatial continuum: From entrance and reception to interior spaces

One of the first issues to face the practitioner (and the patient) is the arrangement of spaces in the office and the traffic flow in and out of these spaces. Often space in our environment is organized in a hierarchical fashion, moving from public to private. This sequence is characteristic of both

Arriving, Waiting, and Taking Vitals **41**

clinically oriented and administratively oriented spaces, which move from the front to the back of the house, so to speak (as illustrated in Figure 2.02).

The public spaces, such as the reception and waiting area(s), are the first to be encountered and are accessible to all users. Moving farther into the setting, passing through a series of transitions and away from the entrance, spaces typically become smaller and more private. We expect this hierarchical organization, based on our expectations/schemas of how these environments, including our own homes, are typically arranged. Figure 2.03 of the Danbury Hospital Pulmonary Department nicely shows how the check-in and waiting areas are encountered first (top of the image) at the "front of house," whereas many of the private spaces, such as the exam rooms, are in the back of the house (bottom of the image). A nice feature of this layout is that the check-out areas are separated from the check-in areas, providing a smooth flow of traffic.

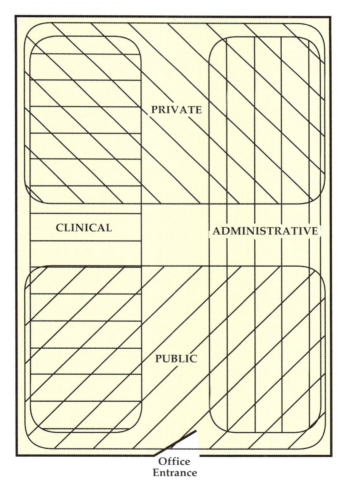

Figure 2.02: *Schematic of public and private, clinical and administrative zones. Illustration credit: Dennis O'Brien, Maps and Wayfinding, LLC*

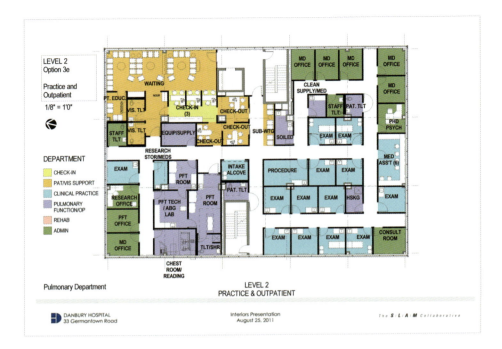

Figure 2.03: *Illustrates a hierarchy of spatial zones, from public to private, particularly check in vs. exam. Location: Western Connecticut Health Network, Pulmonary Relocation, Danbury, Connecticut. Architect and plan: The S/L/A/M Collaborative.*

As explained in Chapter 1, people have schemas, or expectations, about the world they inhabit, based largely on their previous experience with the environment, either directly or through media. Experience in western culture tells us public spaces are in the front of the house; private spaces are reached further into the space through a series of transitions. When people enter the public space at the front of the office they like to assess its possibilities, to see what functions it affords. They assess whether the space matches their schema.

Arrival

The processes of arrival and departure involve interior as well as exterior spaces. These layouts have consequences. You can update furnishings and display new artwork, but changing a spatial layout is complex and expensive. The office layout requires careful consideration, whether you rent and renovate an existing space or deal with new construction. Does the layout support patients so they are not clogged in small hallways? Does the traffic flow in a way that moves from the waiting room, to the station where vital signs are taken, to the exam room without needing to backtrack?[8] In other words, is there a linear progression from reception to waiting, to vital signs with adjacent or nearby restroom, to exam room? This linear progression may seem obvious, but it is far from universal. You want a functional progression of spaces, moving from public to private without backtracking. One example of such an arrangement is seen in Figure 2.04, which reflects the nomenclature of Oscar Newman's defensible space theory. In this theory, the way in which

Arriving, Waiting, and Taking Vitals   43

space is divided can suggest territorial prerogatives.[9] The most obvious examples of such prerogatives are the use of doors to control access.

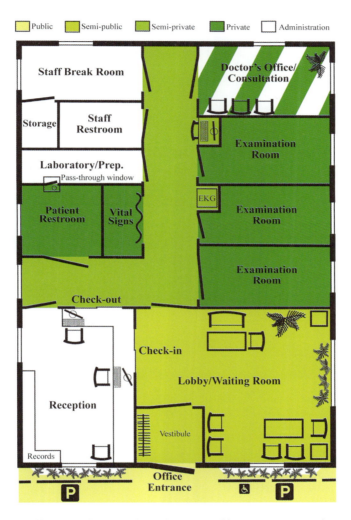

Figure 2.04: *Office layout illustrates the patient's public, semi-public, semiprivate, and private zones. Illustration credit: Dennis O'Brien, Maps and Wayfinding, LLC*

Other advice regarding layout relates to congestion in the hallways and patient traffic. Controlling the number of people in the hallway helps to reduce noise and minimize distractions. Patient privacy is also better protected if there are fewer people in the hallways. In addition, limiting the number of people in the hallway contributes to the impression the office is organized. If some patients visit the office for nonclinical functions (e.g., Lab, Pharmacy), practitioners are advised to place the function at the front of the office suite, as suggested by Figure 2.05, to avoid patients having to pass through more private spaces to reach those facilities.[10]

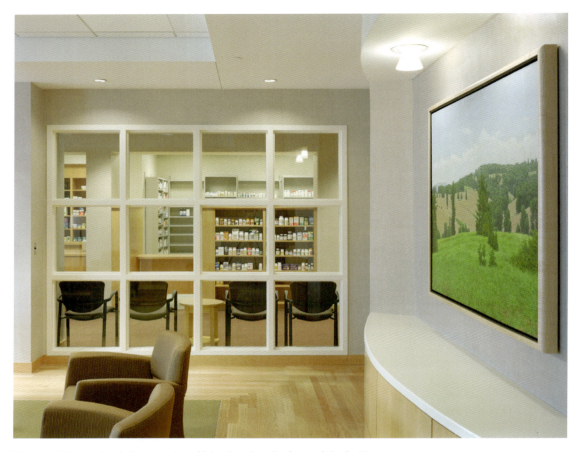

Figure 2.05: *Lab (and pharmacy) could be placed at the front of the facility.*
Location: Lakeland Center for Outpatient Services, St. Joseph, Michigan.
Architect: The S/L/A/M Collaborative.
Photo credit: Woodruff/Brown Architectural Photography

Thinking through how the continuum of public-to-private space is laid out can help practitioners make a first pass at the kind of spatial arrangement desired. Designers will make sure all health and safety regulations are met, but practitioners first need to think about the kinds of spaces they need.

Wayfinding: Navigation cues for patients

In an ideal world, the articulation of the space itself would communicate its function; in other words, a reception space would look like a place where people could check in. In each of the following examples (Figures 2.06, 2.07, 2.08, and 2.09), it is clear from the segmentation of the spaces (Figures 2.06, 2.07, 2.08), and the shape and prominence (2.09) that such interaction is appropriate.

Arriving, Waiting, and Taking Vitals 45

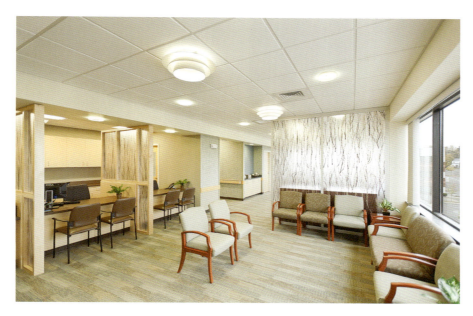

Figure 2.06: *Clear function of space for check in and waiting.*
Location: Greenwich Hospital, Bendheim Cancer Center, Greenwich, Connecticut.
Architect: The S/L/A/M Collaborative.
Photo credit: John Giammatteo

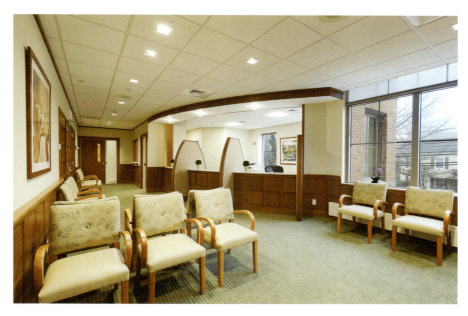

Figure 2.07: *Example of check in with good visual screening between patients.*
Location: Western Connecticut Health Network, Pulmonary Relocation, Danbury, Connecticut.
Architect: The S/L/A/M Collaborative.
Photo credit: John Giammatteo

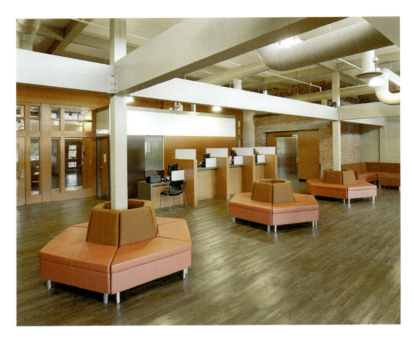

Figure 2.08: *Example of standing check in and nearby seating.*
Location: Thundermist Health Center, West Warwick, Rhode Island.
Architect: Vision 3 Architects.
Photo credit: Aaron Usher III Photography

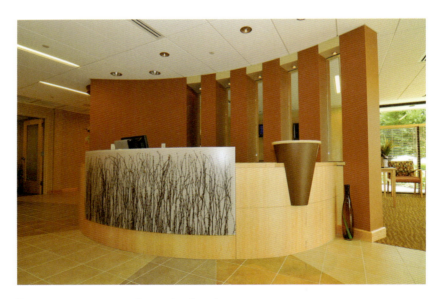

Figure 2.09: *Illustrates transparency of reception function.*
Location: Griffin Hospital, Emergency Department, Derby, Connecticut.
Architect: The S/L/A/M Collaborative.
Photo credit: The S/L/A/M Collaborative

Unfortunately, not all spaces are designed this transparently. The lyrics "You can check out any time you like, But you can never leave!" from the Eagles' song "Hotel California," were mentioned in a colleague's MA thesis. Applied beyond the specific context used in the thesis, these lyrics suggest the "all-too-prevalent habit architects and communication designers have of getting visitors to their destinations with signage and other cues and then letting them figure out how to get back on their own," according to Dennis O'Brien,[11] author of the thesis. This anecdote points to the lack of symmetry in wayfinding. In healthcare settings, it is often easier to find your way to than from a destination. Why? As one architect described this imbalance, the transparency of checking in at a small facility is relatively easy to design (see Figure 2.08). In his words, "It is obvious where to go." Then, a nurse or physician's assistant might escort a patient to an exam room. However, when patients leave the exam room, they often lack an escort. Unless a signage system is provided in addition to whatever degree of transparency the design embodies, patients may not be able to easily retrace their steps.

Many professionals underestimate the importance of wayfinding signage in offices, signage that should be in both English and Spanish. Remember that patients are stressed and anxious about their medical condition. As a consequence, patients may not necessarily mark their wayfinding movements. Sometimes, a building's complexity is a challenge even to those who work there; student nurses who had worked in a complex healthcare facility for a number of months had not mastered the layout.[12] A building's complexity can outweigh the benefits of familiarity.[13]

Manifest and latent cues

What are the kinds of cues that people use to help with navigation? There are two broad categories of cues, manifest and latent. Manifest cues are intended to aid with wayfinding. Typically this is alphanumeric information, consisting of letters and numbers. Latent cues are not specially intended for wayfinding but are relied on nevertheless and are often more successful than their manifest counterparts.[14] An example of using a latent cue is giving the direction to "Turn left by the drinking fountain" or "Use the elevators by the grandfather clock." People often use latent cues to substitute for the inadequacy of manifest cues. If the only distinguishing features in a corridor are the room numbers, people may seek any differentiation to help navigate. Even flooring could be a wayfinding aid, as indicated by these two photographs; one has no differentiation whereas the second at least offers a floor pattern – "look for the hallway with the green floor markings" (see Figure 2.10).

Color as a wayfinding cue: A caution

The latent cue, "Turn left at the red bench" may seem more useful than the manifest cue "Look for Room 206," but even reference to the red bench has a drawback: color. The percentage of people who have the most common type of colorblindness (red-green) is estimated to be about 8 percent of men and 0.4–0.5 percent of women. Color is not routinely noticed as a wayfinding indicator; fewer than 20 percent of residents in a long-term care facility understood that color differentiation was intended as a wayfinding aid.[15] Color by itself is not a reliable wayfinding cue. If color is used as a differentiator, people need to be instructed about its purpose.

To say "Turn left by the grandfather clock" is likely to be useful because of its distinctiveness in the environment. In complex hospital environments, it is fairly common for staff to provide written directions prepared for people to follow. The more successful of these directions include reference to latent cues. Distinctive aspects of the environment (e.g., targeted use of art) in conjunction with a function (e.g., drinking fountain) can assist navigation, as seen in Figure 2.11.

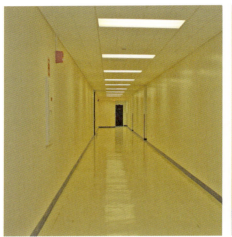 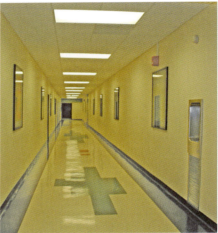

Figure 2.10: *Differentiation added through floor pattern.*
Location: Cummings Arts Center, Connecticut College, New London, Connecticut.

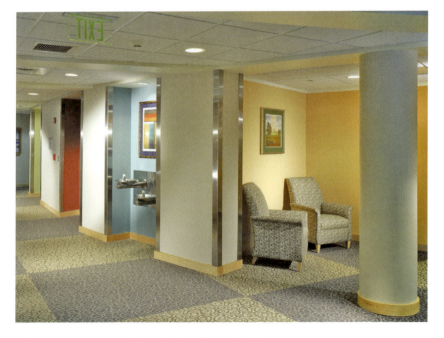

Figure 2.11: *Color in conjunction with landmarks aids wayfinding.*
Location: Lakeland Community Hospital, Niles Michigan.
Architect: The S/L/A/M Collaborative.
Photo credit: Woodruff/Brown Architectural Photography

Arriving, Waiting, and Taking Vitals 49

Use of redundant cues

The adage to repeat information more than once if you want people to remember it applies to wayfinding and can be discussed in the form of redundant cues. Redundant cueing typically means providing information to more than one sensory modality; it can also mean repeating the information more than one time. For example, in an elevator in a medical office building, Braille and auditory signal indicators may be used for each floor, and the floor number can be provided on the floor, literally, usually in contrasting figure-ground tile next to the elevator opening. Using tile rather than carpet at this juncture where everyone stands helps withstand wear and tear, as seen in Figure 2.12.

As the first interior space that is encountered in the practitioner's office, the reception area (which may double as the exit) needs to be evident. Ideally this is accomplished through the design itself (refer to Figure 2.08, for example). The style of the signage should then be repeated throughout the office suite (refer to Figure 1.07); patients will look for a repetition of that style. A number of organizations focus on enhancing visual communication in the built environment, including the Society for Experiential Graphic Design (SEGD); designers may want to consult their website (www.segd.org).

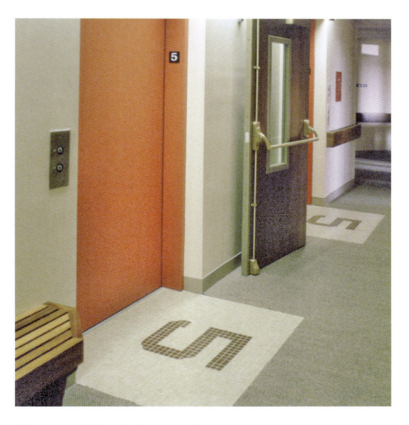

Figure 2.12: *Legibility enhanced through floor numerals.*
Location: Westminster Housing for the Elderly, Providence, Rhode Island.

The view as a wayfinding cue

A view may be a useful latent cue. If you can see out through a window, that vista provides a clue to where you are and where you want to go. In a corridor without windows, you may be lost. As a good example of a simple view that assisted with orientation, a practitioner's office was organized around a center linear spine that ran from the front entrance to the back exit, which emptied into a parking lot. The front door was glass, as was the top half of the back door. The reception area, vital sign area, restroom, and exam rooms were located left or right of the central spine. When a patient came out of an exam room, simply looking left and right clarified which way led to the reception/payment area and which way led to the parking lot. In this more dramatic example in Figure 2.13 from a pediatric hospital in Florence, the transparent walkways constantly remind you of your location with respect to the exterior.

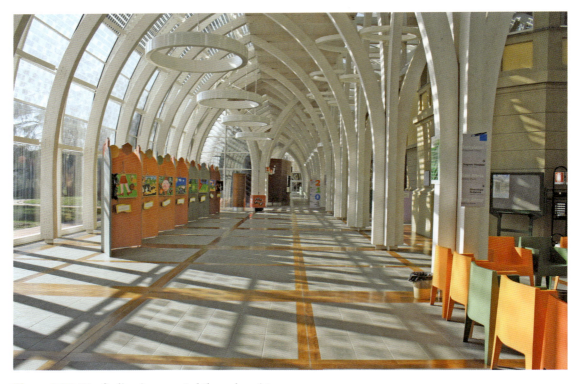

Figure 2.13: *Wayfinding is supported through a vista.* Location: Meyer Children's Hospital, Florence, Italy.

Reception space: Expectations and functions

Our schema of the physician's office is activated as we open the door into the office. When we enter the physician's office we expect to see a reception area because our script is that we need to check in for our appointment. In most solo and small practices, the reception area serves multiple purposes. The reception area often serves as bookends to the visit (checking in and checking out); for most small providers, it is the first and last area of patient contact.

Design can guide patients through the multiple functions the "reception" area may provide. In one example of the division of function in a reception area, a large curved work surface had stations for three separate functions: reception, cashier, and financial aid.[16] The curvilinear nature of this surface with its stations helped patients find the appropriate niche for that part of the visit and spatially separated people making follow-up visits from those who were just checking in. For practitioners with more space, Figure 2.03 depicts spatially separated reception and departure areas where the check-in and check-out functions do not overlap. Even in the small office depicted in Figure 2.04, check in is separated from check out.

Reception windows and counters

In an ideal world, the receptionist would not be separated from the patient by glass, but given auditory privacy issues (calls, conversations, office machines), an acoustical barrier (usually sliding glass windows) is typically necessary. Ideally the receptionist would be able to see all of the patients in the waiting room to help keep track of the flow of patients and to monitor patients who may have mobility issues (e.g., with walkers).

A counter that runs the length of the reception window enables patients to easily fill out forms and make payments. A depth of one foot is adequate and does not protrude too far into the patient reception area. The counter should accommodate people in wheelchairs, which might mean that the counter would have two levels; one for people standing (suggested at 42" off the floor), the other for people sitting in wheelchairs (suggested at 34" off the floor, to comply with ADA specifications).[17]

Check-in stations and kiosks

In most practices, staff members perform the check-in function. In some hospitals, by contrast, automated check-in kiosks, such as the Patient Passport Express™,[18] have been used for a number of years. These automated systems can register and check in patients (note their arrival, provide the opportunity to update insurance information) and check out patients (collect co-payments, schedule follow-up tests and future appointments, as necessary). Some facilities, even in relatively small offices, have begun using computer check-in systems, which come in a variety of sizes, from freestanding (like an ATM) to a tablet. From the standpoint of practice management, it is possible to use such systems to check on the current status of insurance information; future appointments can also be noted. The collection of co-payments is more reliable with this system, according to the CEO of Connected Technology Solutions, which markets Patient Passport Express™.[19] Another benefit, according to some users, is to provide something for patients to do as they wait for their appointments. These systems also provide the opportunity for targeted advertising, which may appeal to some providers and potentially generate revenue.

Reception area and HIPAA concerns

The relationship of computer screens in the receptionists' area to patient check in and check out can be problematic, in particular the visibility of patient records to those who are checking in. Some practitioners may want to consider use of a computer privacy screen, which can be easily installed to eliminate visibility of information on the screen from anyone looking from an angle. Looking from the side, onlookers would see only a darkened screen; this technology is readily available from such companies as 3M. The most problematic design aspect is the protection of information on the screen when looked at head on by unauthorized viewers. Thus, computer screens are best located beneath the check-in window on the side where the receptionist sits, as is the case in the left image of Figure 2.14; in this location screens are not visible to patients checking in. Similarly, patient information should not be visible to others when patients exit. In the right image of Figure 2.14, the large opening is the patient check out, with the monitor appropriately facing toward staff (the opening also seems to "frame" the art on the wall of the corridor). Both photographs were taken from the same staff area.

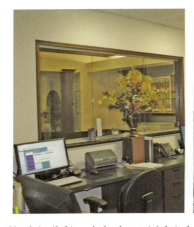 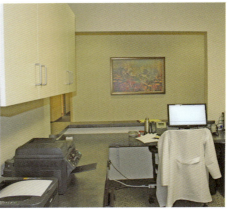

Figure 2.14: *Check in (left) and check out (right) show monitor position facing away from patients, supporting patient confidentiality.*
Location: Office of Neeraj Kohli, MD MBA, Wellesley, Massachusetts.

To demonstrate the lengths to which patients' information is safeguarded, Griffin Hospital uses separate cubicles for patient registration, seen in Figure 2.15).

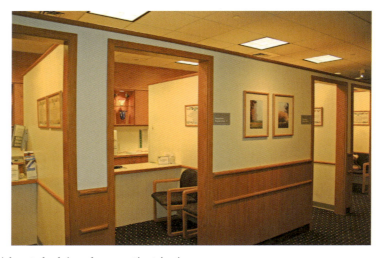

Figure 2.15: *Cubicles at check in enhance patients' privacy.*
Location: Griffin Hospital, Derby, Connecticut.

Arriving, Waiting, and Taking Vitals

The waiting room: Territoriality, personal space, and privacy

Waiting rooms have been described as "soulless spaces with sterile, cold qualities, that remind us of illness rather than wellness,"[20] but they need not be. Waiting rooms are essentially way stations between arriving and consulting with a doctor. Research indicates that the average waiting time in a doctor's office is 23 minutes.[21] As bad as sitting in a waiting room may be, sitting alone in an exam room may be worse; at least the waiting room typically has positive distractions. One customer service strategy adopted by the Lucile Packard Children's Hospital at Stanford is not to send patients to an exam room until a practitioner can actually see them.[22] At Yale-New Haven Health System, another healthcare facility featured in Press Ganey's best practices report, a second area of customer improvement was cultural sensitivity, which was enhanced by offering consent forms and other information in as many as 14 different languages through a computer-based system.[23]

Patients may feel possessive about spaces in the waiting room. Their reactions influence the degree of comfort felt in the setting. Formally, the psychological concepts used to describe such perceived spatial control and the psychological states it affords are territoriality and personal space (the regulation mechanisms) and privacy (the state we may desire to varying degrees).

The environmental psychologist Irwin Altman defined privacy as the "selective control of access to the self or to one's group."[24] In Altman's model, territoriality and personal space are mechanisms of interpersonal control that influence whether the degree of privacy we desire is achieved. The pivotal concept in design is choice. If privacy is desired, are there seating choices on a continuum ranging from fairly isolated from others to adjacent to others, as is shown in Figure 2.16? These options can be created through the clustering and arrangement of seating groups, as this waiting area shows.

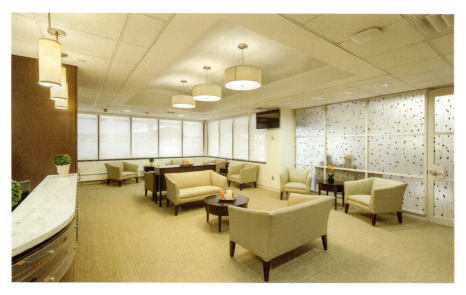

Figure 2.16: *Clear choice of seating options.*
Location: Clara Maass Medical Center, Continuing Care Building, Cancer Center Reception, Belleville, New Jersey.
Architect: The S/L/A/M Collaborative.
Photo credit: John Giammatteo

The degree of territoriality established relates to the regulation of privacy. When the Adult Emergency Room waiting area at Yale-New Haven Hospital was renovated, seating groupings were created that provide a great deal of choice for patients (see Figure 2.17). Noteworthy also is the absence of television in this waiting area (television use is discussed in detail in Chapter 4). The presence of television was perceived to signal that "a long wait is ahead of you" – a message the hospital did not want to send.

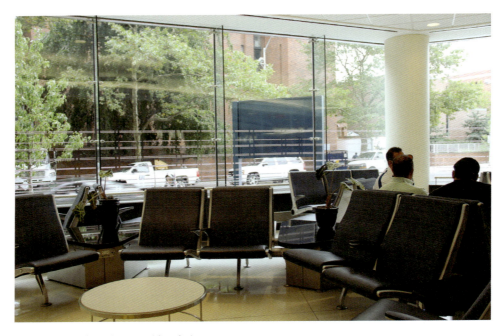

Figure 2.17: *Clustered seating provides choices.*
Location: Yale-New Haven Hospital Adult Emergency Waiting Area, New Haven, Connecticut.

Territoriality

Territories can be broken down into the categories of primary, secondary, and tertiary, or public.[25] Primary territories are those, like the doctor's personal office, essentially under the owner's exclusive control. Secondary territories have some degree of perceived ownership (e.g., the seat you always select for a class you are taking), but whatever control you have is temporary. In the context of the doctor's office, an exam room, once you are occupying it, is a kind of secondary territory. Tertiary or public territories are equal access, open to everyone; waiting rooms fall into this category.

Claiming a seat is one of the few acts of control patients have within the waiting room. The goal is to have enough seats to provide choice, but not so many that people feel lost in the space (and may wonder about the success of the practice when so few patients are waiting). Langer and Rodin's often-cited research showed that selecting a plant and tending to it (rather than relegating those decisions to staff) was associated with better behavioral and health outcomes, such as active participation in activities, for the elderly in a nursing home.[26] Having the opportunity to actually choose where to sit is a form of control, as is being able to adjust a table lamp.

Personal space

Personal space is a virtual spatial regulation mechanism, sometimes called a bubble. Personal space moves with us and regulates our degree of comfort with interpersonal distance, which is how close others are to us. When people with whom we have no personal relationship come too close to us, we feel psychological discomfort. Seminal research on this topic is associated with E. T. Hall, whose book *The Hidden Dimension*[27] covers proxemics (the study of how space and culture are related). Hall identifies four zones of interpersonal distance: intimate distance (0–1.5 feet), personal distance (1.5–4 feet), social distance (4–12 feet), and public distance (greater than 12 feet). Seating preferences are related to personal space norms. Unless there are no other seats available, most people will not sit next to another person. Think about the last time you were sitting in a movie theater and someone sat right next to you when other seats were available. This behavior violates a social norm about respecting personal space.[28] The level of discomfort in these kinds of spatial intrusions may lead to departure; you may get up and move.

Normally, the spatial zone between touching someone to about 18 inches away is reserved for intimate relationships;[29] in the doctor's office we allow strangers to be that close to us if no other seats are available. This accommodation happens through furniture. Furniture helps regulate spatial behavior and essentially permits an increase in density (the number of people in the given space) by providing solid boundaries (e.g., chair arms), allowing more strangers to be at ease in the setting than without such boundaries.

To help establish clear personal space boundaries, waiting room chairs with arms are preferred to armless chairs, as Figures 2.18 and 2.19 illustrate.

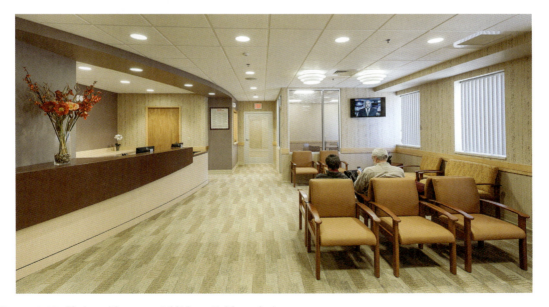

Figure 2.18: *Chairs with arms establish spatial boundaries.*
Location: Western Connecticut Health Network, Breast Imaging Renovation, Danbury, Connecticut.
Architect: The S/L/A/M Collaborative.
Photo credit: John Giammatteo

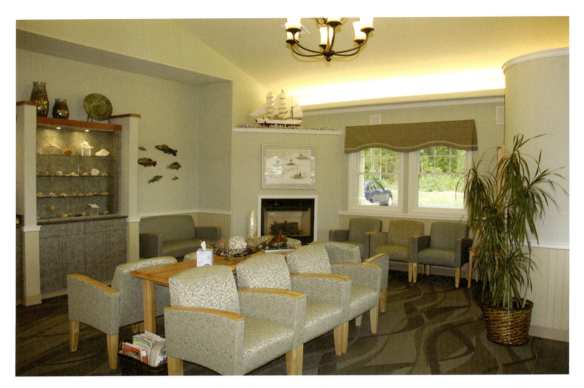

Figure 2.19: *Bariatric seating is among the needed seating options. Location: Coastal Connecticut Dentistry, Waterford, Connecticut.*

Chairs with arms have the additional benefit of providing support for older people who may need a stable platform to push up to a standing position. Another recommendation is to provide seating for patients who are heavy; such bariatric seating typically has a sturdy back and wide seat. For some obese patients a chair without arms may be appropriate because it more easily accommodates their frame.[30] Healthcare furniture manufacturers now provide a range of these bariatric seating choices to accommodate those who are large, as is evident in the seating next to the fireplace in Figure 2.19. The wide seating in this dentist's office could also be used for two family members – for example, a parent and child. Patients have different needs, and the waiting room should provide choices – choices in the size of chairs; choices in where to sit.

Seating and social interaction

Early research showed that sitting side by side, as in the typical waiting room, inhibits social interaction;[31] but is social interaction desirable? Some people may want to engage in conversation, especially if family members or friends have accompanied them, but most do not. Seating arrangements should allow people to avoid the gaze of others if they wish; in other words, people do not want to be forced to sit directly across from someone in close proximity.

From an evolutionary standpoint, humans desire both prospect (a vista) and refuge (a place of retreat). In terms of seating arrangements, people typically want to sit with their backs against a

Arriving, Waiting, and Taking Vitals

wall or at least against a divider. At the same time, practitioners will want to avoid lining up all chairs against the wall, which someone has labeled "the doctor's waiting room" effect[32] (partly suggested by two walls in Figure 2.20). In this particular room, having windows makes the chair arrangement tolerable. The bariatric chair on the far right in this picture also provides a welcoming option.

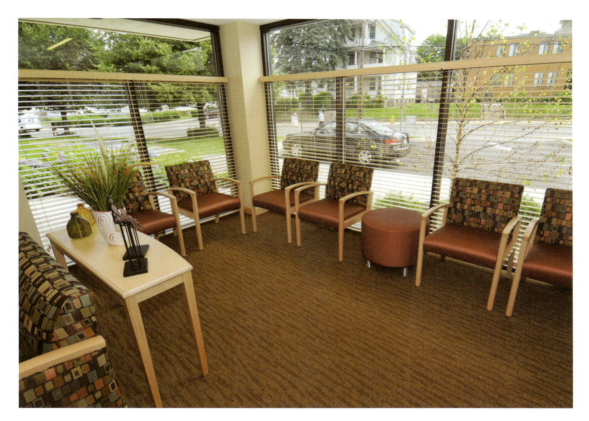

Figure 2.20: *Windows soften the "doctor's waiting room" effect.*
Location: Griffin Hospital, Emergency Department, Derby, Connecticut.
Architect: The S/L/A/M Collaborative.
Photo credit: The S/L/A/M Collaborative

To avoid the doctor's waiting room effect, a small number of chairs can be clustered in groups.[33] You might have a series of small groupings in different parts of the room using tables as a focus (visible in Figures 2.16 and 2.17) or a series of small semicircles. Whatever pattern is selected, care must be taken to make sure that people in wheelchairs and walkers can maneuver through the paths that have been created with these groupings. To help create clusters, practitioners can use acoustic separators[34] – acoustically insulated panels that provide space for private phone calls, which inevitably occur given the length of time people may wait. Such dividers now support technology, which increasingly plays a role in passing the time of waiting, as shown in Figure 2.21

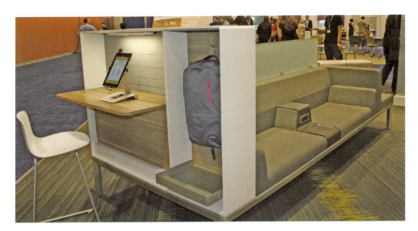

Figure 2.21: *Support for technology is an increasing part of the waiting experience.*
Location: 2012 Healthcare Design conference, Phoenix, Arizona.

This furniture, the Regard™ line for Nurture® by Steelcase was introduced at the 2012 Healthcare Design Conference and won a gold Nightingale award for guest seating.

Even in waiting rooms with expensive furnishings, researchers at Cornell commented that seating arrangements needed more attention.[35] Furnishings can be expensive without being comfortable or being arranged comfortably. In their research, what psychologist Robert Sommer has called soft architecture[36] was positively received. Settings that embody soft architecture typically have furnishings with padded furniture, personalization, carpeting, and soft lighting, as evident in the waiting area in Figure 2.22.

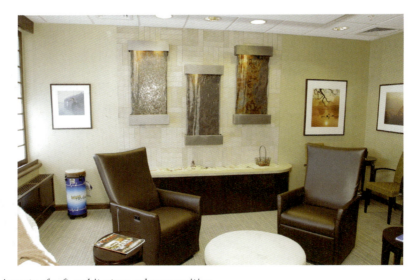

Figure 2.22: *Aspects of soft architecture enhance waiting.*
Location: The Ken Hamilton Caregivers Center at Northern Westchester Hospital, Mount Kisco, New York.
Architect: The S/L/A/M Collaborative.
Photo credit: Northern Westchester Hospital

How many seats do you need?

One consultant says you can estimate the number of seats you will need in the waiting room by thinking about how many patients a doctor sees in an hour (e.g., 6). You need to account for family and friends by multiplying the number of patients by 1.5 to 2.5 (yielding 9 to 15 seats). Next, subtract the number of patients who would occupy exam rooms at any given time (e.g., 3, for 3 exam rooms). This subtraction (9 − 3 or 15 − 3) yields 6 to 12 places to sit. If you multiply the number of chairs by 20 square feet, it yields the square footage needed for the waiting room.[37] Similarly, in her text on space planning for medical and dental facilities, Malkin provides a similar formula: "2P x D − E = S, where P = Average number of patients per hour per physician, D = Number of physicians, E = Number of exam rooms, S = Seating." She suggests the multiplier 18 square feet per person, with extra allowances for wheelchairs.[38] Consultants who help create physicians' office spaces should check local codes to verify how wide pathways need to be; the turning radius of wheelchairs; doorway width; and accessibility for toilet rooms and counters.[39] As a note, having too many seats may feel uncomfortable but having too few is worse, both in terms of a perception of crowding (i.e., the feeling that there are too few seats for the number of people) and in the lack of available choice.

Opportunities for personal control

Personal control is a psychological concept dealing with the perceived ability to manipulate the environment; it is associated with competency motivation, the idea that humans like to be effective.[40] Any step that can be taken to reduce the sense of powerlessness that patients feel should be considered. Waiting encourages a sense of powerlessness and is experienced throughout the visit, from arrival to departure.[41] What parts of this process are within patients' control? Typically, not many. Patients have a lack of control over how long they wait, and perceptions of longer waiting times are generally more negatively associated with quality of care ratings than are perceptions of shorter waiting times.[42]

Having personal control over the physical environment has been associated with positive outcomes.[43] The theory of supported design suggests that healthcare environments will promote well-being if they are designed to foster: 1) sense of control over physical-social surroundings, 2) access to social support, and 3) access to positive distractions.[44] In this chapter we focus on control over the physical environment. In the waiting room, practitioners can provide a number of ways for patients to exert some control.

Being able to choose where to sit, to adjust lighting, to select magazines, and to access Wi-Fi, are examples of such control. Incorporating accessible technology is appearing even in healthcare furnishings, as Figure 2.23, taken at the 2012 Healthcare Design Conference, illustrates. There are power outlets in this seating, the Regard™ line for Nurture® by Steelcase.

Over 50 percent of Americans use the Internet to search for health information, but the percentage e-mailing their doctors is only 5 percent.[45] When patients search the Internet for health information, digital patient communities arise in which patients communicate with each other about their disease. Providing a computer for patient use in the waiting room to research health issues might open an avenue for communication with patients. Furniture is being designed to accommodate such technology and provide seating for using it (seen in Figures 2.21 and 2.23).

In addition to choosing where to sit (discussed in an earlier section), patients should have the opportunity to control task lighting consistent with whatever activity they select (e.g., reading). To provide this degree of control, the waiting area needs enough end tables with lamps and enough current reading material, either on the tables, on shelves, or in magazine racks near each cluster of seating, as Figures 2.24 and 2.25 nicely demonstrate. Racks or shelves provide the opportunity to keep materials organized.

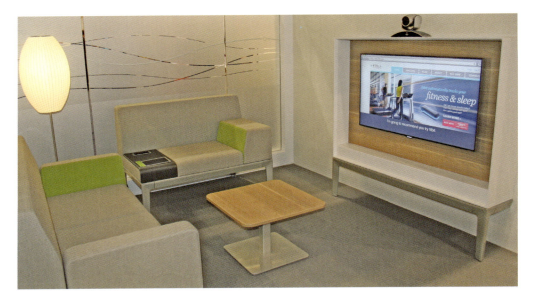

Figure 2.23: *Power sources incorporated into furnishings.*
Location: 2012 Healthcare Design Conference, Phoenix Arizona.

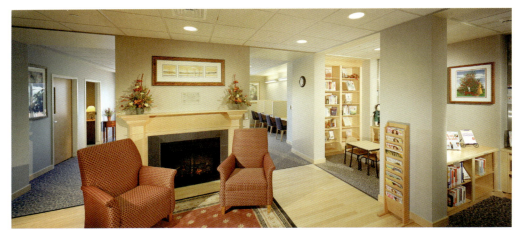

Figure 2.24: *Residential furnishings and storage support reading.*
Location: Lakeland Community Hospital, Niles, Michigan.
Architect: The S/L/A/M Collaborative.
Photo credit: Woodruff/Brown Architectural Photography

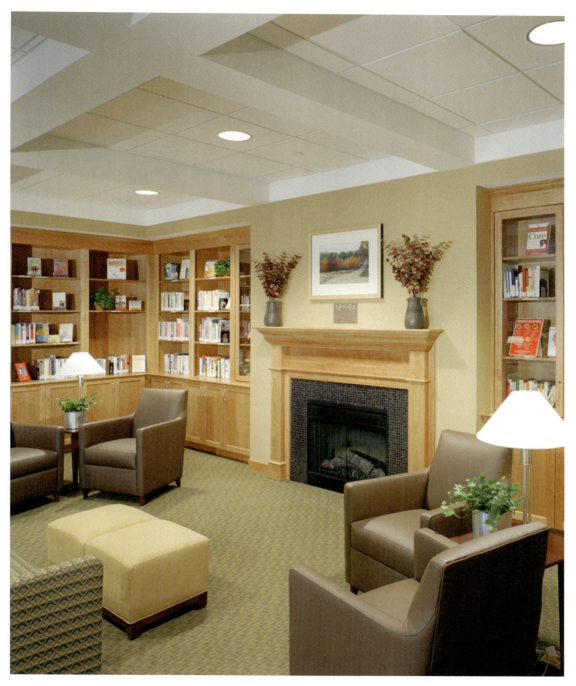

Figure 2.25: *Residential task lighting supports reading.*
Location: Lakeland Center for Outpatient Services, St. Joseph, Michigan.
Architect: The S/L/A/M Collaborative.
Photo credit: Woodruff/Brown Architectural Photography

Lighting

Personal control

There may be overhead lighting, but task lighting of a residential nature is desirable (refer to Figure 2.25). Having table lamps on end tables where people might sit and read provides the opportunity to exert some degree of control. Such lighting should be adjustable (low, medium, high), and larger-size switches are available to accommodate patients with arthritis or other impairments in mobility of the hands. If the medical practice serves a majority of elderly patients and/or patients with limitations in the use of their hands, lamps that are pressure sensitive, called touch lamps, are recommended.

Functions

Related to lighting, there are multiple activities occurring in a waiting room; these include movement through the space, but also stasis, which typically means sitting and waiting. Given these needs, lighting sources must address multiple functions. The amount of light (the number of lumens emitted by a source) needed for reading will be different from that needed for movement (walking through the waiting room). Lighting has different visual properties, in addition to its ability to illuminate. For example, incandescent is softer than fluorescent; but enough lighting has to be provided for sure footing as patients move across the room. Where possible, natural light should be a major element in the design. Further, adjustments should be part of every lighting source, whether controlling sunlight through the use of blinds as seen in Figure 2.26, or adjusting the number of lumens through settings on a table lamp. Every seating grouping for four to five patients needs an end table or a small table to accommodate a lamp; such groupings have the advantage of dividing up the waiting room space to create small territories. Both overhead and task lighting are important.

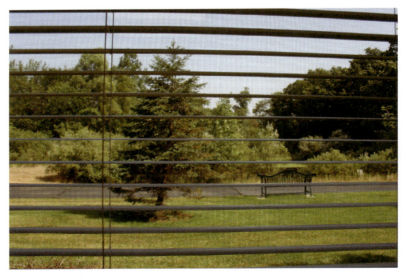

Figure 2.26: *Use of blinds to control glare.*
Location: Towsley Village Memory Care Center, Chelsea, Michigan.

Types of lighting

Full(er)-spectrum lighting simulates the visible and ultraviolet (UV) spectrum of natural light, although sunlight is the only true full-spectrum lighting. Numerous health benefits have been associated with full-spectrum lighting, but causality has not been verified. In research on office environments, fatigue was reduced and alertness increased when bulbs that are fuller spectrum, more like sunlight, replaced the fluorescent bulbs typically used.[46] In healthcare settings, having more sunlight (46 percent more than those in shaded rooms) was associated with reports of less pain and less stress; these patients with more sunlight also used 22 percent less pain medication.[47] These reports suggest that both full-spectrum lighting and natural lighting are beneficial in the practitioner's office.

Furnishings

The movement in healthcare settings toward hospitality and customer service can be seen in the kinds of furnishings selected, many possessing qualities of soft architecture. A white paper with an extensive bibliography from the Center for Health Design provides an evidence-based design checklist for furniture design and healthcare outcomes. Typical recommendations are for surfaces that are easily cleaned and nonporous; moreover, furnishings should not have volatile organic compounds (VOCs) (e.g., formaldehyde). At the same time, noninstitutional appearance is important.[48] Among the recommendations is avoiding sharp edges on chairs or tables to prevent injuries if patients fall. Fabrics that meet these criteria are surprisingly noninstitutional in appearance, as the display of colorful fabrics in Figure 2.27, at the 2012 Healthcare Design Conference, demonstrates.

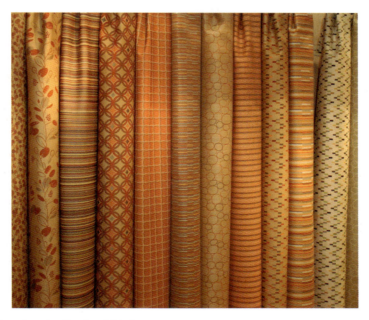

Figure 2.27: *Colorful and noninstitutional fabrics.*
Location: 2012 Healthcare Design Conference, Phoenix, Arizona.

The variable of choice plays a role in furnishings as it has elsewhere. Not only is the location of the chair relevant to patients but the type of seating is as well, as was previously discussed. High-backed seating will accommodate older patients and those with back problems. With regard to upholstery, Malkin notes the wide variety of durable fabrics available that do not shout "institutional." She recommends using a blended fabric combining nylon with a natural or synthetic fiber and provides a list of manufacturers, including Designtex, Arc-Com, and Sina Pearson Textiles. Manufacturers' specifications relating to durability, lightfastness, staining, and flammability should be considered.[49]

Such leading furniture manufacturers as Herman Miller (which acquired Nemschoff in 2009) and Steelcase have developed product lines targeted for healthcare environments. With regard to lounge seating, Nemschoff provides a range of seating widths and shapes to create a comfortable experience while waiting.[50] The fabric choices include nonwoven upholstery (vinyls, polyurethanes, silicone), impermeable woven upholstery (surface-treated with antimicrobial agents), and woven upholstery treated to withstand discoloration and fading.[51]

Nurture® by Steelcase is a product line of furnishings designed for healthcare environments and lists as its partners the American Academy of Healthcare Interior Designers, The Center for Health Design, and the Planetree Organization, among others. "Today's waiting room is far more than a place to sit and wait. It has to support activities and needs for privacy, work, technology, education and relaxation. Seating has to accommodate people of all sizes...."[52] The furnishings activate a schema for a hotel lobby or café. Steelcase recommends accommodating groups of different sizes by clustering different types of seating and offering amenities, such as workstations and refreshments, which help people maximize their time[53] (see Figure 2.21 as an example). Beyond its own research, Steelcase is an external partner to the Mayo Clinic[54] in the SPARC innovation program – See, Plan, Act, Refine, Communicate. Launched in 2004, the program has already brought innovation to the design of the healthcare environment.

The scaffolding functions: Staff preparation and storage areas

A useful way to think about the differences between physician and staff areas is that those for staff provide the scaffolding to make medical procedures possible. Therefore, the administrative areas, storage areas, and clinical preparation areas are important to seamless functioning in the medical office.

Practitioners may employ two types of staff: administrative and clinical. Administrative staff members are generally in the "front" of the house and handle such functions as patient check in, check out, billing, insurance, and scheduling. There is typically a barrier, literally and figuratively, between administrative staff and patients (refer to Figures 2.04 and 2.14). Practitioners are now making the transition from paper to electronic records. Until that process is complete, space savers may include collapsible shelving.

Arriving, Waiting, and Taking Vitals 65

Vital signs, nursing station, and location

In a nursing station, clinical staff perform a variety of functions, from assessing vital signs to giving injections, dispensing drug samples, and performing lab tests considered routine.[55] The size of the space and its location will vary with the extent of the activities performed there. Increasingly, the design of spaces for procedures and medical equipment emphasizes screening, to avoid reminding patients of procedures. Doors that screen medical equipment and waste are becoming more common, as seen in Figure 2.28, in which large doors screen equipment and drugs that might be used.

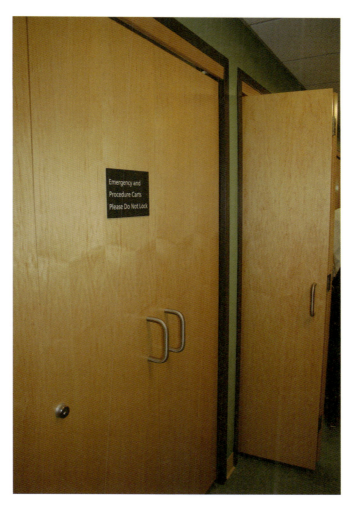

Figure 2.28: *Doors screen equipment.*
Location: Neonatal Intensive Care Unit of the Women & Infants Hospital of Rhode Island, Providence, Rhode Island.

In the sequence of public to private space, a small space for assessing vital signs is often located in what could be categorized as semiprivate space, where there is some but not complete control of access. One model for vital signs that is frequently used is a small alcove or recess, approximately 4' x 6', on the corridor that leads from the waiting room to exam and consultation rooms. In this space there is a chair for patients, a scale, and a shelf (see Figures 2.29, left image, and 2.04) and/or hooks for a stethoscope, blood pressure cuff, and thermometer. In the office of a solo practitioner or small group practice where only one patient may be served at a time, the open alcove method may suffice. For larger group practices, it is important that the opening into the corridor be offset from access to the waiting room or check-in function; in other words, care must be taken for some visual screening. In the image on the right in Figure 2.29, a translucent screen was added post occupancy because the area where patients were weighed (now behind the screen to the left of the EXIT sign) had been visible to patients checking in. Figure 2.30 shows a larger area with a privacy screen for vital signs and other procedures. If the alcove model is used, a nursing station for supplies and more involved procedures must still be provided.

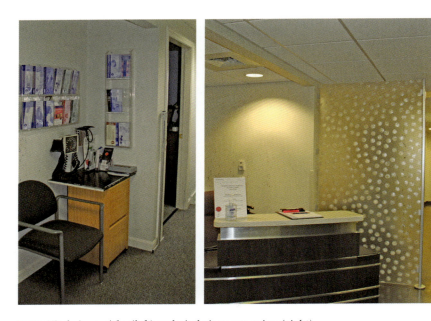

Figure 2.29: *Vital signs niche (left) and vital signs screening (right).*
Location: Office of Timothy Barczak, MD, New London, Connecticut (left); Women & Infants Center for Reproduction and Infertility, Providence, Rhode Island (right).

In the second model, a wider range of procedures is performed in a single nursing station area, and a larger space is required (e.g., 8' x 12'),[56] both for the procedures themselves and the supplies required. If blood is drawn (phlebotomy) in this area, the room should accommodate full visual and auditory privacy; that is, a door or doors that could be closed, as seen in Figure 2.31. The location of this larger nursing area might be closer to the exam or consultation rooms rather than on a corridor where there is a lot of traffic. Whatever model is used, attention should be given to the décor here, just as in other areas of the suite. There is wall space for positive distractions such as artwork or a floral touch on the windowsill.

Arriving, Waiting, and Taking Vitals 67

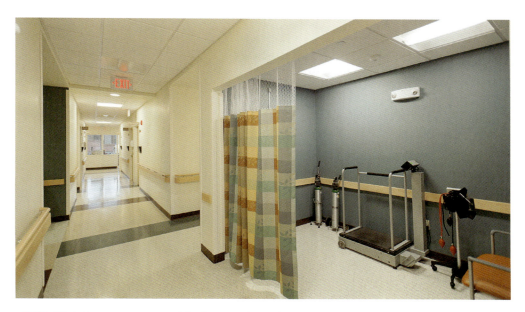

Figure 2.30: *Vital signs area accommodates large equipment.*
Location: Western Connecticut Health Network, Pulmonary Relocation, Danbury, Connecticut.
Architect: The S/L/A/M Collaborative.
Photo credit: John Giammatteo

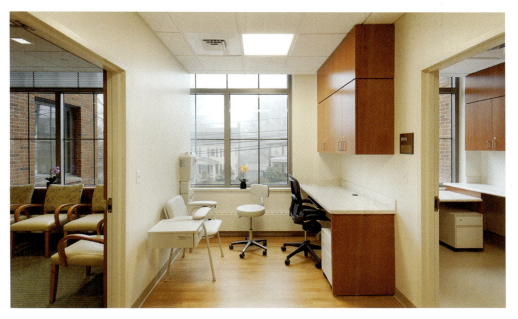

Figure 2.31: *Area for phlebotomy with doors that can be closed for privacy.*
Location: Greenwich Hospital, Bendheim Cancer Center, Greenwich, Connecticut.
Architect: The S/L/A/M Collaborative.
Photo credit: John Giammatteo

Laboratory functions and traffic flow

Often in a small practice, a small lab space exists to perform urinalysis and other routine tests, as seen in Figure 2.32; but if the practice is one in which laboratory functions might be performed without a clinical visit (i.e., if people might come solely for labs), traffic flow to and from the lab is a consideration (refer to Figure 2.05).

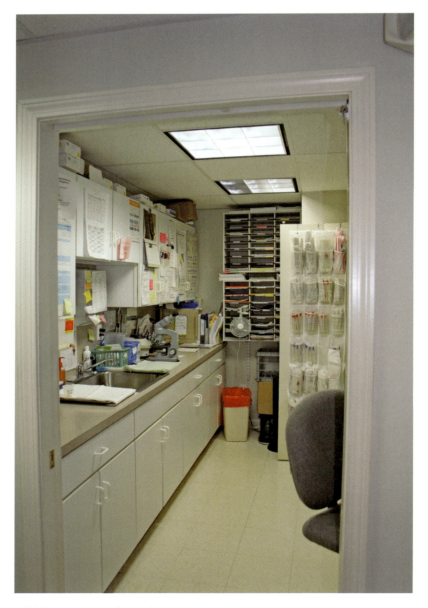

Figure 2.32: *Small laboratory space for onsite analysis.*
Location: Office of Timothy Barczak, MD, New London, Connecticut.

Locating the lab nearer the front of the office suite will limit the invasion of private spaces and reduce traffic flow into the interior spaces.[57] The reception area might serve both laboratory and clinical patients, but the waiting room/area, clinical support area for vital signs, and exam and consultation rooms would be located in spatial zones further into the suite than the location of the lab.

Staff areas

Communication: Implications for patient privacy

Staff members need the actual support space to assess patient functioning and store the equipment for these measurements. The locations of these spaces need to be carefully considered with regard to what patients and others could hear. When patients overheard conversations about medical status, had their own body parts exposed to others, or saw the body parts of others, they were less likely to share their own health information with staff than when no privacy breaches occurred.[58] These findings from an emergency room should inform decisions about where staff work areas are located in a practitioner's office. A walled rather than a curtained cubicle reduced the likelihood of experiencing a privacy violation.

Designing space to protect patients' privacy involves all aspects of the practitioner's office – from HIPAA concerns about check in, to conversations overheard in hallways, to who passes by an open door into an exam room. Not infrequently, one sees signs like: "Remember patient information should not be discussed in public areas," which was posted in elevators at the University of Michigan Medical Center. Not only does noise interfere with concentration, but also the transmission of speech threatens privacy. For those reasons, considering the spatial layout of functions and using sound absorbing materials for ceilings and walls, especially in exam areas and rooms, is recommended.[59]

Staff lounge and toilet areas

Drawing on the culture of correctional facilities, there's a saying that the staff do more time than the inmates. Staff members are present the entire workweek, and areas where staff can take breaks, eat lunch, and use toilet facilities separate from patients are recommended. Hamilton and Shepley[60] emphasize the importance of spaces for staff that provide relief from stress, such as spaces with a view, ideally with elements of nature visible as in Figures 2.33 (top image), which is preferable to a space without windows (bottom image). If the space and site permit, a terrace or courtyard is welcome. The staff toilet could be located adjacent to the staff lounge.

The recommendations from a critical care unit are useful in the context of the doctor's office. Such spaces should be welcoming and separate from the spaces used by patients and visitors; appliances such as refrigerators and microwaves are recommended (refer to Figure 2.33), as is sufficient seating to relax.[61] Given the popularity of single-cup coffee brewers, such a machine might be a good addition to a lounge, especially because it provides an opportunity for control and choice. You personally select your beverage. Malkin notes that having staff areas for eating keeps eating out of areas where sterility is a concern.[62] In her view, if the practice has three or more employees, a lounge is warranted but need not be large (perhaps 10' x 12'). In addition,

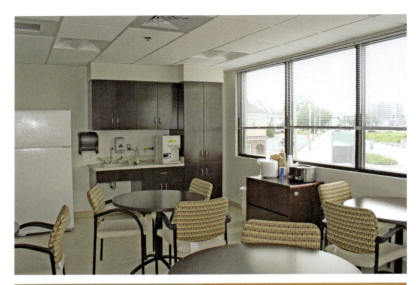

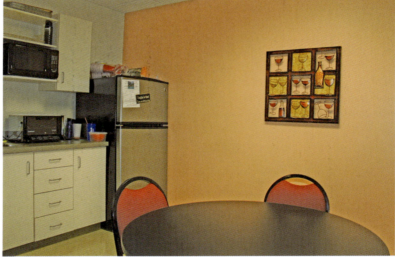

Figure 2.33: *Attractive staff lounge spaces.*
Location: Women & Infants Center for Reproduction and Infertility, Providence, Rhode Island (top); Office of Neeraj Kohli, MD MBA, Wellesley, Massachusetts (bottom).

Malkin reminds us that a refrigerator with an ice maker necessitates a water line.[63] Providing a storage area for staff belongings is also important; using attractive lockers is one solution.

Supply and storage functions

Medical practices all deal with supplies for procedures and medication, and for cleaning and disposal of waste. The supplies for procedures and those for cleaning could coexist in the same room, with adjustable shelving dedicated for each function. Storage can certainly communicate

Arriving, Waiting, and Taking Vitals 71

aesthetic values. The disposal of waste should be separated. If there is a small room for soiled linen, the biomedical waste can be stored there until picked up by a licensed disposal company; this area has to be secured and the waste has to be clearly labeled.[64] Such waste is picked up by a licensed firm once a month or more frequently, depending on the practice volume. In Figure 2.34, supplies for procedures as well as brochures are stored in a large, lighted closet accessible to nursing staff along the hallway adjacent to patient rooms.

Ideally, a storage area would be located adjacent to the nursing station, where a more limited range of supplies is kept on hand for procedures. The storage area should be farther away from patient areas than it is from the nursing station and close to the receiving area where supplies are delivered, often at the back of the office suite near the parking area. The size of the practice will dictate the square footage needed.[65] The small, labeled, secured storage area for medical waste would be close to the receiving area in a place where patients would not view its transport.

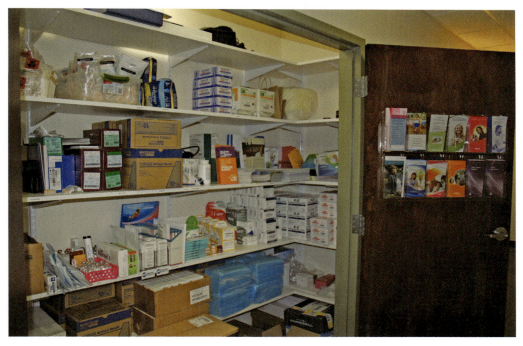

Figure 2.34: *Convenient corridor storage.*
Location: Office of Neeraj Kohli, MD MBA, Wellesley, Massachusetts.

The toilet room (restroom)

First, a comment about nomenclature. Technically, the room where people provide urine specimens and excrete waste is a toilet room, which includes a toilet and sink. Most people call this space a restroom or bathroom, and patients would be used to seeing the room labeled as a restroom or simply with the international symbols associated with that purpose. Here, the words restroom and bathroom will be used.

We guarantee privacy for elimination in our culture, which places very specific demands on the layout of the office. An important compendium of information is Alexander Kira's *The Bathroom*, in which he states: "as almost anyone who has ever had to provide a urine specimen can testify, modesty and privacy play a big role in our ability to perform."[66] Anxiety surrounds having to ask about the location of the restroom. Kira describes this request as giving up privacy to obtain privacy.

In the case of the medical office and restroom use, patients' whereabouts are known, but they desire not being seen or heard.[67] For that reason, sound-proofing in restrooms is important. Kira describes the concern with "privacy-from" others as opposed to "privacy-for" the individual.

The quality of the patient's bathroom is a reflection of overall quality, claims Malkin, noting that hotel bathrooms are used as a similar benchmark of quality for those establishments.[68] Similarly, Kira describes the image of the host that is created by the bathroom.[69] In talking about the differences in priorities of a gas station owner and a restaurant owner with regard to the restroom image, Kira notes that in a Triple A survey of drivers' complaints, dirty restrooms are second only to poor directional signing. In other words, restrooms and their condition matter. To the extent that the environment reflects care, the patient may come away with the sense that someone understands the dehumanizing aspects of the process. To elevate the quality of the patient's experience, such facilities must combine utility with residential décor (see Figures 2.35 and 2.36).

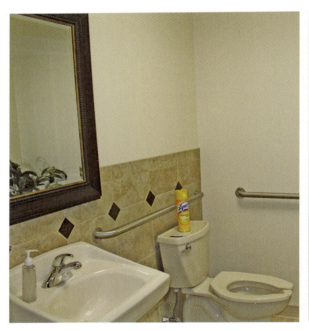
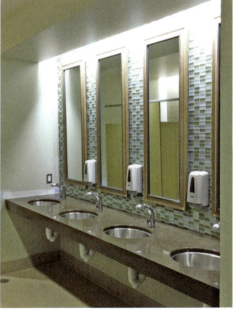

Figure 2.35: *Use of decorative tile to enhance appearance.*
Location: *Office of Neeraj Kohli, MD MBA, Wellesley, Massachusetts (left); UPMC East, Monroeville, Pennsylvania (right).*
Architect: *BBH Design and IDeA (right).*
Photo credit (right): *Maggie Dillon, IDeA*

Arriving, Waiting, and Taking Vitals

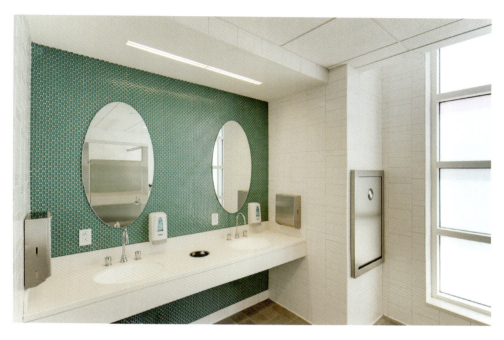

Figure 2.36: *Colorful tile backsplash brightens the space.*
Location: Northern Westchester Hospital, Emergency Department, Mount Kisco, New York.
Architect: The S/L/A/M Collaborative.
Photo credit: John Giammatteo

Patients, staff, or both? Public? Private? The restroom locations

Who are the primary users? Are there secondary users? In other words, is the restroom dedicated to patients? Might staff use it as well? For reasons of providing patients with privacy and control, and separating the roles of staff and patient, a minimum of two restrooms is warranted. The location of the staff restroom is an easier decision than is the location of the patient restroom(s). The staff restroom would be located in the private zone of the office suite, presumably at the end of a corridor where patients have no reason to be. To provide the necessary visual and auditory privacy for staff, the restroom for staff should not open onto their break room or lounge (refer to Figure 2.04), nor should it be adjacent to the restroom used by patients.[70]

Patients' restrooms: Private office location vs. public corridor

Providing a restroom (with that label) in the waiting area has the advantage of convenience to waiting patients (and visitors) during the wait before the formal exam commences and makes good sense in pediatric practices.[71] A restroom for patients would still be needed in the more private spatial zone of the exam rooms.

This question of where to locate restrooms is more easily resolved in the design of medical office buildings with public restrooms on each floor. People who are accompanying patients, or patients visiting physicians where needing to provide a urine specimen is essentially nil (e.g., orthopedics, ophthalmology), can use the restroom before entering the office suite. A restroom for patients would still be located in the suite, but it could be within the more private spatial zone.

Number of restrooms: Individual occupancy

For a solo practitioner, the single-user restroom makes a great deal of functional and economic sense. Occupied one person at a time, it can be labeled to accommodate individuals of any gender, eliminating the need to provide separate restrooms labeled by gender, which is no longer a matter of restrooms for men or for women. Gender-neutral restrooms, accommodating those who identify as transgendered, are necessary. Two or more solo-occupancy, gender-neutral restrooms, side by side, may make sense. If toileting functions are a more pronounced part of the practice, as is the case in OB-GYN medicine, consideration should be given to: 1) increasing the number of restrooms, and 2) locating these rooms near the nursing station to make use of the specimen pass-through as the mode of specimen delivery.[72]

Protocol for leaving the specimen

When patients are asked to leave a urine specimen, the analysis is accomplished either using a chemical dipstick on site or being transported for thorough analysis in a laboratory. There are three models of transferring the specimen for urinalysis. Patients can: 1) leave the specimen in the restroom, 2) hand the specimen to the nurse or physician's assistant, or 3) use a specimen pass-through provided in the restroom.

Where is the specimen left in the restroom? Some practitioners provide a tray that sits on the top of the toilet tank; others provide a table, typically across from the toilet, where the specimen(s) can be left. Both of these approaches are somewhat awkward in my view. The specimen pass-through, the most professional option, works best when the nursing station or lab is adjacent to the restroom (refer to Figure 2.04).

Maintenance, storage, and functionality

In a restroom for a medical practice, the demand for cleanliness may exceed what one might expect in a public restroom because people are providing urine samples. Women may actually soil a toilet more than do men, given women are often taught never to touch the seat and as a consequence may spray urine outside of the toilet bowl when voiding.[73]

The supplies required are paper towels, toilet and facial tissues, and hand sanitizers. In the context of an OB-GYN practice, Malkin[74] mentions the need for hooks to hang coats and handbags, a shelf, and a waste container for sanitary products such as feminine napkins and tampons. These recommendations are valid across medical practices. Putting a hook on the back of the door is one efficient way to deal with the need to hang up belongings.

With regard to storage, the restroom could contain a closet, either built-in or freestanding, for storage of toilet paper, paper towels, soap dispenser refills, specimen cups, grease pencils, and light bulbs. Alternatively, this closet could be located in the corridor adjacent to the restroom. If the supplies are kept in the restroom, the cabinet should be locked or otherwise un-openable by children.

Paper towels are still preferable to warm air dryers and jet air dryers in terms of drying efficiency, bacterial growth, and the spread of bacteria in the environment.[75] Paper towels are also "quiet." With paper towels and other waste, care must still be taken to screen the discards. What that requires is a canister with a swing top or cover with foot pedal, rather than an open rim in which the discards would be visible.

Lighting

Recommendations for patients' bathrooms in hospitals can be applied to the doctor's office. With regard to lighting, Malkin notes that lighting above a mirror can make people look less healthy because of the shadows cast; for that reason she recommends lighting on both sides of the mirror.[76] Attention should also be given to avoid glare. The color of the light bulbs is relevant as bulbs that provide fuller spectrum are preferred in terms of making people look healthier.

Positive distractions and aesthetics

Reading materials in the restroom may be provided for distraction and relaxation. With regard to color, a band of decorative tiles can break up the monotony of and add color to an otherwise homogeneous restroom; ceramic tile with a pattern is another way to create visual variety[77] (refer to Figures 2.35 and 2.36). Artwork can also be displayed in the restroom to provide positive distraction.

Further Reading

Arneill, Allison B., and Ann Sloan Devlin. "Perceived Quality of Care: The Influence of the Waiting Room Environment." *Journal of Environmental Psychology* 22 (2002): 345–360. doi:10.1006/jevp.2002.0274

Becker, Franklin, and Stephanie Douglass. "The Ecology of the Patient Visit: Physical Attractiveness, Waiting Times, and Perceived Quality of Care." *Journal of Ambulatory Care Management* 31, (2008): 128–141. doi:10.1097/01.JAC.0000314703.34795.44

Hamilton, D. Kirk, and Mardelle McCuskey Shepley. *Design for Critical Care: An Evidence-Based Approach.* New York: Architectural Press, 2010.

Herczeg, Laszlo. "It's Not Just about Time. A Fuelfor Design Exploration into the Experience of Waiting in Heathcare." Barcelona: Fuelfor, 2011. http://issuu.com/fuelfor/docs/waitbook_pdf/8?e3264945/3977126

Kira, Alexander. *The Bathroom.* New York: The Viking Press, 1976.

Leather, Phil, Diane Beale, Angeli Santos, Janine Watts, and Laura Lee. "Outcomes of Environmental Appraisal of Different Hospital Waiting Areas." *Environment and Behavior* 35, (2003): 842–869. doi:10.1177/0013916503254777

Malkin, Jain. *Medical and Dental Space Planning: A Comprehensive Guide to Design, Equipment, and Clinical Procedures*, 3rd ed. New York: John Wiley & Sons, Inc., 2002.

Malkin, Jain. *A Visual Reference for Evidence-Based Design.* Concord, CA: The Center for Health Design, 2008.

Ulrich, Roger S. "Effects of Interior Design on Wellness: Theory and Recent Scientific Research." *Journal of Health Care Interior Design* 3, (1991): 97–109.

Consultation and Examination Spaces: 3
"You Feel Healthier When You're Dressed"

Overview

"You feel healthier when you're dressed."[1] This comment from a patient at the Mayo Clinic reflects the importance of control to the patient, in this case of bodily privacy. In this chapter on exam and consultation spaces, opportunities to enhance patient control are described. Seligman's learned helplessness theory[2] suggests we become hopeless and helpless when we believe we cannot control outcomes; the design of exam and consultation spaces can return some control to patients. Two types of spaces are described in this chapter: the exam room, where traditional physical exams are performed, and the consultation space, where practitioners confer with patients. These spaces can be separate or the exam room can serve both functions.

Anxiety and the medical consultation

Almost half the information patients hear is forgotten; moreover, the more information presented, the lower the proportion recalled correctly.[3] With the impact of anxiety on retention,[4] we can see how important it is to help patients feel less anxious, especially when the information concerns a life-threatening medical condition. Most attempts to increase recall focus on the medium of presentation (e.g., audio recordings, written materials, visual aids) or strategies used, either cognitive (e.g., rehearsal) or interpersonal (e.g., personalized teaching).[5] The physical environment is overlooked. How can patients feel more in control and less anxious in consultation and exam spaces?

Models of consultation

There are two general models of exams, which typically involve physical assessment or palpation. One model gives more control to the patient. In this model, the visit begins in a consultation space where the patient remains clothed. In a small office practice, the consultation might occur in the doctor's own office (refer to Figure 2.04). Then the patient moves to an exam room, often adjacent to the doctor's office. Here the patient dons a gown and undergoes the physical exam; blood work and/or an EKG may be performed. Next the patient dresses and returns to the doctor's office where further consultation (assessment of status, prescriptions, discussion of follow-up tests) occurs. In the second model, all of these functions are performed in the examination room and the patient is fully clothed much less of the time. For that reason alone, using separate consultation and exam spaces is desirable to give patients more control.

The traditional exam room

In a typical internal medicine practice with four physicians, there may be four offices (one for each physician) and five exam rooms; three doctors may practice on any given day, rotating between two exam spaces. The exam rooms are laid out in the same fashion to facilitate the rotation. Exam rooms range from about 8' x 10' to 10' x 12' with the exam table in the center, often at an angle; the patient's head typically faces away from the door. If there is a window, shades or blinds are drawn during patient exams, and about 3 feet into the room or in a corner of the room a privacy curtain is often suspended from the ceiling. This curtain, seen in image 3.01 and the right image of Figure 3.02, can be pulled closed to shield the patient when the door is open, although this step may be neglected. Screening can also be used to provide a visual barrier when entering an area with a number of patients' rooms, as shown in the left image of Figure 3.02.

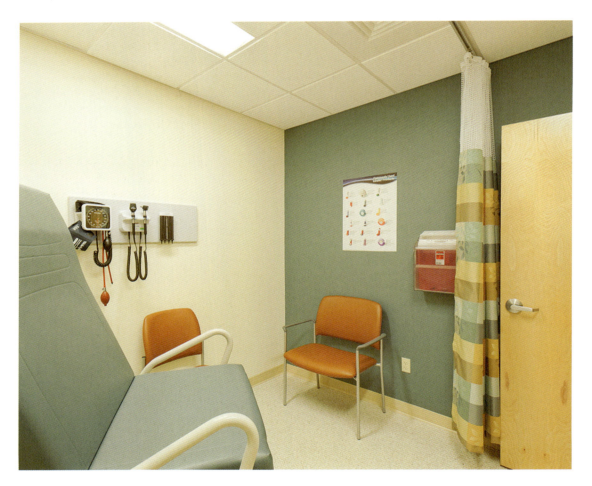

Figure 3.01: *Screening using a colorful cubicle curtain.*
Location: Western Connecticut Health Network, Pulmonary Relocation, Danbury, Connecticut.
Architect: The S/L/A/M Collaborataive.
Photo credit: John Giammatteo

Consultation and Examination Spaces 79

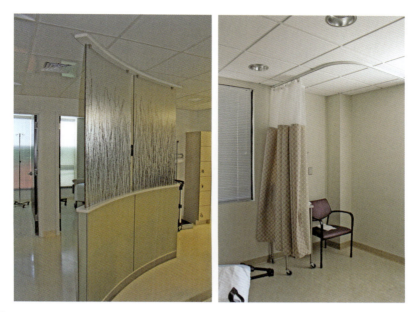

Figure 3.02: *Screening occurs both prior to (left) and within the exam room (right).*
Location (left and right): Women & Infants Center for Reproduction and Infertility, Providence, Rhode Island.

A sink is typically part of a workspace with cabinets, as shown in Figures 3.03 and 3.04. Such rooms accommodate a chair and/or stool, a small mobile equipment cart, a wall-mounted rack for the pressure cuff, stethoscope, pocket-size otoscope and ophthalmoscope, and an exam light.

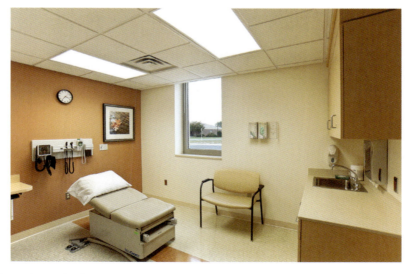

Figure 3.03: *Art, color, and cabinetry enhance this functional exam space.*
Location: Onslow Hospital, Radiation Oncology Center, Jacksonville, North Carolina.
Architect: The S/L/A/M Collaborative.
Photo credit: John Giammatteo

80 Consultation and Examination Spaces

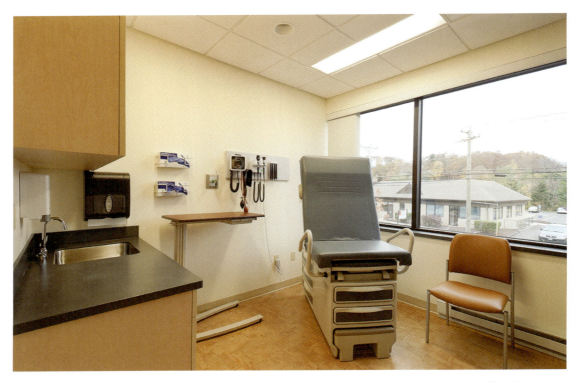

Figure 3.04: *The wall-mounted rack, glove boxes, sink, paper towels, and hand sanitizer support clinical functions.*
Location: Western Connecticut Health Network, Pulmonary Relocation, Danbury, Connecticut.
Architect: The S/L/A/M Collaborative.
Photo credit: John Giammatteo

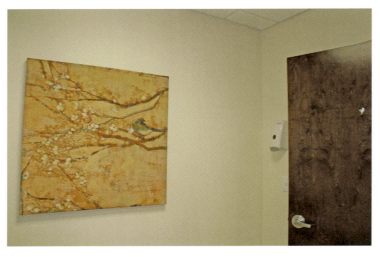

Figure 3.05: *Small (often-overlooked) features, such as a door hook for clothing, support patient-centered care.*
Location: Office of Neeraj Kohli, MD MBA, Wellesley, Massachusetts.

Consultation and Examination Spaces

Hazardous waste is stored separately from other waste. The chair may be used for patients to lay their clothing after undressing for the exam, although some practitioners with foresight install wall or door hooks. A wall-mounted hand sanitizer on the side of the door may greet you as you enter and/or exit the room. In addition, there may be artwork (e.g., posters, watercolors). In Figure 3.05, both the hand sanitizer and artwork are visible, as is a hook on the back of the exam room door. In small group or solo practices, the EKG cart may move between patient rooms and the hallway, often its resting location, as seen in the hallway niche in Figure 2.04.

Exam room layouts

There are choices in the layout of the exam room (e.g., which direction the exam table faces; where the sink is located; where any family seating is positioned); each layout has benefits and drawbacks. Cahnman provides models of four different rooms (see Figure 3.06)[6] that illustrate some of the trade-offs. Room A offers patient privacy because the patient is facing away from the door, without an obvious need for a cubicle curtain; but the sink placement makes it somewhat less accessible to the clinical zone, she says. In Exam Room B, a cubicle curtain is required to safeguard patient privacy given that the exam table is perpendicular to the entry. Another issue in this model is locating family seating in the back of the room, which may interfere with the clinical tasks. In Exam Room C, with the exam table directly facing the door, patient privacy again needs to be safeguarded with a cubicle curtain, but an advantage is the location of the sink relative to the clinical area; the family seating in the front half of the room is also farther from the clinical zone. The larger room, Exam Room D, provides both the consultation and exam room in one space, separated by a partition. If desired, family members could also be accommodated in the consultation area during an exam. Cahnman says the layout in Exam Room D is more typical of private facilities abroad (Europe, Middle East, Asia) than in the United States.

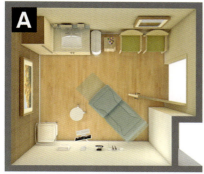
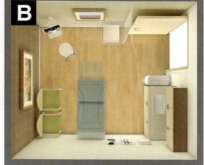
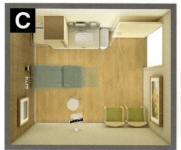
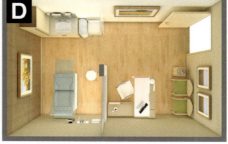

Figure 3.06: *Possible exam room layouts. Illustration credit: Sheila F. Cahnman, AIA, ACHA, former Group Vice President, HOK. Credit: Reprinted from* Health Facilities Management *by permission, June 2011, Copyright 2011, by Health Forum, Inc.*

There might be different solutions for different kinds of practices, especially when patients bring a variety of cultural expectations. If we emphasize patient privacy, we typically put the patient zone deeper into the space of the room (reflecting our understanding of spatial hierarchies). We may need (and need to use) a privacy curtain to manage patient privacy in the front of the room.

"Having a seat at the table"

How might this typical layout be improved? Patients increasingly bring health-related information, often downloaded from the Internet, to their exams. If consultation occurs in the exam room, the practitioner needs a space where the patient can display this information. This need to display information and the seating to discuss it is transforming how consultation space is designed.

In one collaboration between the Mayo Clinic and Steelcase, reported at an EDRA conference,[7] a semicircular table was constructed and tested to provide adjacent seating for patients and practitioners. Patients displayed their printed-out Internet searches on the table, and practitioners uploaded the medical records on a plasma screen mounted on the table. What the designers had not anticipated was just how favorable both clients and physicians would be about this new work surface, in particular because it brought physicians to the level of the patients. Patients and physicians were literally and figuratively at the same table. Published research on this intervention used a randomized controlled trial comparing a standard consultation space with this experimental room (the semicircular table where the computer monitor was equally visible and accessible to patients and physicians). The results showed a significant impact on patients of the computer monitor's equal availability around the semi-circular table: being able to better interact with the monitor, see their medical information, and have the clinician review the medical record more than was true of the standard arrangement. At the same time, there was no significant difference in patients' satisfaction with the consultation, mutual respect, or the quality of the communication that transpired.[8] Nevertheless, in my judgment any design step that increases the ability of patients to have better access to their medical information in the context of the consultation is important to incorporate.

The Jack-and-Jill layout

The Mayo Clinic has a tradition of innovation in healthcare delivery. This innovation is apparent in the design of a suite of rooms referred to as the Jack-and-Jill rooms.[9] In their book *Outside In: The Power of Putting Customers at the Center of Your Business*, Harley Manning and Kerry Bodine[10] describe how designers at the Mayo Clinic's Center for Innovation considered what kinds of changes could be made in an exam room configuration that had been the standard for 100 years. As Manning and Bodine describe, after building a foam board mock-up and testing reactions over a two-month period, designers realized a new configuration, separating exam from consultation space, was needed.

In outpatient facilities in a new building, limited space prevented constructing enough exam room/consultation pairings for all clinicians. This limitation led to the breakthrough idea, called a "Jack and Jill," based on the bathroom/bedroom layout in "The Brady Bunch" television series. The bathroom in the television series had two doors, one from each flanking bedroom (one for girls, one for boys). In the healthcare setting, the exam room with doors on either side is usable by doctors consulting with patients in flanking consultation spaces. Research and observation at the

Consultation and Examination Spaces

Mayo Clinic revealed that much of what occurred in an examination was communication, without use of medical instruments. For that reason, fewer exam rooms and more consultation (and less expensive) spaces might suffice.

Testing also suggested brighter lighting and a slightly higher temperature was needed in the exam than consultation rooms. When patients returned to the consultation space, nursing staff could efficiently clean the exam room – a benefit of the Jack-and-Jill arrangement, note Manning and Bodine. Similarly, when patients went into the exam room, family members could remain in the consultation space. If the patient desired, the door between exam and consultation space could be left slightly open to enable family members to hear the patient and doctor exchange.

Location of consultation and exam spaces

Multiple exam rooms can be arranged in different configurations. The row is common, but grouping rooms in a pod has some advantages. In a pod organization, "exam rooms are arranged so a nurse in the central location can see every exam room door. The physician goes from room to room, working in a continuous circle."[11] This arrangement maximizes productivity. The nurse is the key driver of efficiency in this model; when patients leave the room, the nurse gives them "the doctor's instructions, cleans the rooms, moves a new patient in and places the chart outside the door."[12] The physician may use whatever exam room is available, rather than a dedicated space. Standardization of the rooms permits physicians to predict the location of instruments. In the linear (row) model, a single loaded corridor may reduce space needs, but visibility of what is occurring along the row may be reduced.

The exam room: Same-handed vs. mirror image

The healthcare industry lags behind other industries (e.g., aviation) in combating human error where risks are high.[13] To reduce errors, standardization in the physical environment is now being embraced in healthcare. One current debate is between same-handed vs. mirror image inpatient rooms. In same-handed rooms, the headboard is always in the same position as you enter (typically to the left as caregivers are taught to approach from the patient's right side). In mirror-image rooms, the headboard faces the same shared wall from one room to the next (i.e., one to the left, the next to the right as you enter the room). Same-handed rooms are more expensive to construct because the column with the plumbing pipes (the plumbing chase) is not shared between rooms.[14] In same-handed rooms, benefits have been reported in patients' quality of sleep, fewer near falls, and nurses' satisfaction with how the space at the patients' bedside was organized.[15] The trend is toward same-handed rooms, recognizing that such familiarity decreases errors as staff members know where to look for equipment, but more research on the topic is warranted.[16]

In the case of the exam rooms in a practitioner's office, same-handed rooms also make sense. If you want to find things, you need to put them in the same place, every day; that is where you look for them.[17] In the exam room, these "things" include permanent installations such as the sinks, privacy curtain, hand sanitizer, light switches, data jacks, and power outlets. Movable items such as gloves, ophthalmoscopes, blood pressure cuffs, and thermometers need a storage location as does the technology for EMRs. Figures 3.03 and 3.04 show wall racks to store equipment and wall-mounted glove boxes. Storage for other supplies and portable equipment must be provided as well.[18] Microsoft provides templates for exam room layouts that give practitioners the opportunity to concretely think about where functions are located within the room.[19]

Shared functions

One controversy, discussed in an article about office redesign, is eliminating the sink in exam rooms and instead having a central nursing station with a number of sinks to serve all the rooms. The advantages are a gain in counter space and a decrease in plumbing costs, but this approach is not universally embraced. A designer quoted in the article points to our theme of patients' expectations and schemas: "Patients expect sinks in the exam room and expect to see doctors wash their hands …. The patient needs to see it. It is a visual cue."[20]

Another idea about sharing in the clinic setting is "hotelling," a concept from the workspace literature.[21] In hotelling, workers have no permanently assigned workstation or computer and instead register for a workspace, as they would a hotel room (hence the label). In the case of healthcare, hotelling typically applies to spaces with technology that are essentially interchangeable. Patient information (e.g., EMRs) can be updated on a monitor available in a nook shared by a number of staff. In the example in Figure 3.07 from a NICU at Women & Infants Hospital of Rhode Island, a workstation niche is provided between two patient rooms.

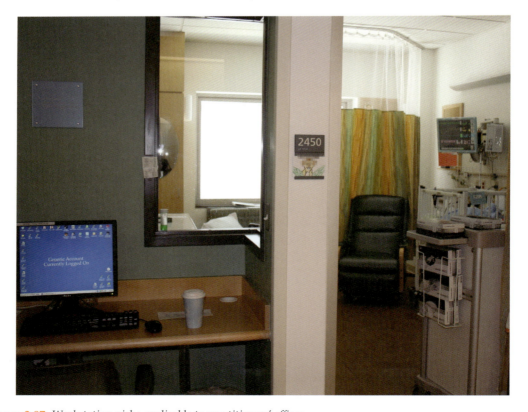

Figure 3.07: *Workstation niche applicable to practitioners' offices.*
Location: Neonatal Intensive Care Unit of the Women & Infants Hospital of Rhode Island, Providence, Rhode Island.

Consultation and Examination Spaces 85

This idea could be adopted along the corridor of patient rooms in a practitioner's office, ambulatory care, or community health center (see the niche for the computer station in Figure 2.04).

In an approach that required a change of culture, Thundermist Health Center in West Warwick, Rhode Island abandoned private offices and instead uses a large shared space that flattens the medical hierarchy (see Figure 3.08). The room takes the place of private physicians' offices and traditional nurse stations and is a space where staff can go to do paperwork and informally consult about cases in a confidential setting, according to the project designers, Vision 3 Architects.[22] Preliminary reports suggest this shared space has worked well, but it involves a substantial change in traditional medical culture. To what extent this arrangement is generalizable is unknown.

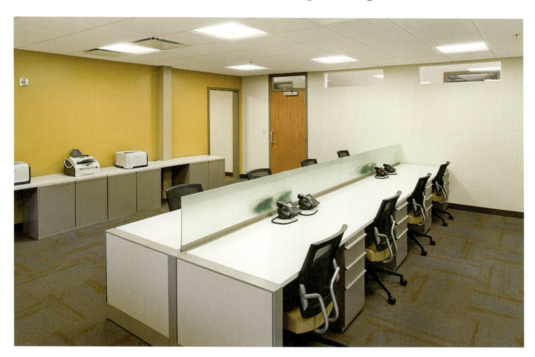

Figure 3.08: *Group workspace supporting all medical staff.*
Location: Thundermist Health Center, West Warwick, Rhode Island.
Architect: Vision 3 Architects.
Photo credit: Aaron Usher III Photography

Functional aspects of the exam room
Undressing and privacy

The fact that patients disrobe in an exam room needs more attention in design. A privacy curtain, when provided, can be pulled across the area screening the door (refer to Figures 3.01 and 3.02, right image). A colorful curtain with a design (refer to Figure 3.01) provides the chance to humanize the room and is a form of positive distraction. Consider the pattern of any curtains in the room and the cubicle drape fabric as these provide the opportunity to enhance the décor.

To provide more choice and control for patients, a dressing area, nook, or alcove should be available for patients to hang their clothes. If a clearly labeled small closet with hangers or hooks cannot be provided, a hook on the back of the exam room door could be used. Expecting patients to drape their clothing over a chair reflects insufficient concern for patients' dignity.

Clutter, waste, and infection control in the exam room

Waste management is an important issue in medicine with particular emphasis on the disposal of hazardous wastes and "sharps." Exam rooms will have a container for the disposal of sharps (e.g., disposable needles) to be discarded after an injection is given or blood is drawn. Once full, these containers are typically placed in a storage area in the suite and picked up on a weekly, biweekly, or monthly basis, depending on the number of patients served in the practice. In addition to this receptacle, at least one other waste container is typically present in the exam room.

Consideration should be given to screening the trash and linen hamper if cloth gowns are used. Often the waste receptacle for non-hazardous waste is simply a plastic wastebasket with a disposable liner. However, it is possible to borrow ideas for screening trash in hospital rooms and adapt them to the practitioner's office.[23] The linen hamper and trash can be completely out of view; they can be screened (see Figure 3.09). In this example, the trash is accommodated through using a pull-out drawer.

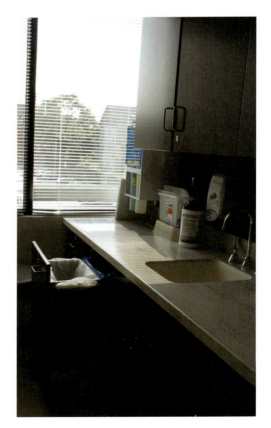

Figure 3.09: *Pull-out drawer neatly screens medical waste. Location: Women & Infants Center for Reproduction and Infertility, Providence, Rhode Island.*

This screening mirrors what was recommended for the early practitioner's slop jar, water basin, and pitcher in 1905. Many recommendations from 100 years ago, such as the screening of hygiene functions, make good sense; yet, until quite recently, the design of medical facilities has not recognized their value. For the last half century, the accommodation of technology has taken precedence over reducing patients' anxiety. These early writers recognized that the screening of sanitation/hygiene functions had a positive impact on patients.

To avoid infection and contamination, one designer recommends restocking the exam room frequently with gowns, linens, and other supplies and storing the bulk of these items in a central storage space.[24] One practitioner uses a supply closet convenient to a corridor of patient rooms for many of these items (refer to Figure 2.34).

Privacy concerns: Overview

"Privacy protection may arguably be one of the defining issues of our time,"[25] whether we are talking about an office or healthcare environment. This protection comes to the fore in HIPAA considerations that deal with EMRs, but conversations that occur anywhere in the healthcare suite can compromise patient privacy. Typically HIPAA considerations concern the spoken and written word, but a case can be made that visual privacy, specifically viewing the patient partially dressed or in an examination gown, is a violation of the person's privacy and dignity.

Auditory privacy

In hospital environments, there is a good deal of concern about noise levels; noise interferes with concentration and the communication of medical information. In the office suite, too little sound is a problem as well. Problems may occur when there is insufficient background noise to mask conversations in exam spaces, consultation spaces, administrative spaces, and hallways.[26] When people had their conversations overheard in an emergency department (and in research 36 percent of them did), they were less likely to share information with staff.[27] The principle of protecting privacy applies to the hierarchy of spaces, from the more public like the waiting room to the more private like the exam room.

An issue paper from the Center for Health Design[28] notes that noise, speech privacy, speech intelligibility, and music all impact members of the healthcare community. Speech privacy is "how well a private conversation can be overheard by an unintended listener."[29] For practitioners' offices, applicable principles include installing sound-absorbing ceiling tiles and reducing staff conversations, and, if used, replacing overhead paging systems with noiseless paging technology. In the issue paper, the major advantage to the sound-absorbing tiles is the reduction of sound reverberation and propagation, rather than absolute decibel levels.

In the exam rooms themselves, the issue paper recommends walls that extend up to the deck to prevent sounds from passing to adjoining exam rooms. The authors observe that walls in such spaces often stop at the ceiling, thus permitting sound transmission. Also, when non-absorbing ceilings are installed, they note sound can pass from one room to another through the plenum. With regard to another way to deal with speech privacy – sound masking – the authors acknowledge that more research on the topic is needed in healthcare settings, which differ in many ways from open-plan commercial offices.

To control noise in the healthcare environment, a research summary from Herman Miller Healthcare suggests focusing first on walls.[30] The report notes that 70–80 percent of the acoustical properties in the patient's room are accounted for by properties of the floor and ceiling. Acoustical tiles and sound-absorbing carpet can be used without diminishing the properties of infection control and cleanliness.[31] These guidelines are reasonable to apply to the practitioner's office.

Nurses impact patients' privacy, including the pattern of private information being divulged in public spaces such as hallways.[32] As researchers point out, these violations are behavioral; but they may be related to design issues, such as having an insufficient number of places to retreat for discussion of confidential information. Moreover, when computer screens are not attended, both other staff and patients have the opportunity to access information inappropriately. Places where such information may be inappropriately shared included waiting rooms, computer screens left unattended, and telephone conversations conducted where they can be overheard.[33]

If the purpose is to mask human speech, one recommendation is to use a sound-management system. A sound-masking machine (also known as a white noise machine) is recommended rather than machines that introduce sounds of the natural environment (e.g., waves or rain) because these machines are specifically designed to mask human speech and are more effective for that purpose.[34] However, if your goal is to change the environmental ambiance, you may want to introduce nature sounds or soft music (a topic covered in Chapter 4). Another recommendation is to put the white noise emitter in the room where the sound will be heard (i.e., for the listeners), not in the room where the sounds will be produced.[35]

The HIPAA regulations do not require structural changes to facilities. The guiding principle is the notion of taking reasonable safeguards, which is a repeated phrase in the regulations. Physicians are permitted, for example, to call out patients' names in the waiting room. At the same time, structuring the environment to minimize the need to call out a patient's name seems a step toward treating patients with greater dignity.[36] The most distracting form of sound is speech;[37] in addition, discussing a patient's condition within earshot of others poses a threat to patient privacy and is a violation of the HIPAA guidelines.

The Acoustic Environment Technical Brief (Green Guide for Health Care™) provides a series of guidelines that are useful in considering materials in the healthcare office. For doctors' offices and exam rooms, dBA levels are 35–45; for conference rooms, 30–40 dBA. To reduce sound, small changes include putting padding in the bottom of patient chart holders outside exam rooms and using folded paper towels instead of rolled towel dispensers.[38]

Beyond using sound absorbing materials, other aspects of the environment can be adjusted to reduce sound. Extending research done in intensive care and general hospitals and suggestions made by Hilton,[39] one could close doors where appropriate, turn down the volume on telephones, and dim the lights, which is associated with people lowering their voices. In addition, education of both staff and visitors can address reductions in noise and simultaneously increase speech privacy when people are reminded not to talk loudly in a healthcare environment.[40] The admonition, "Remember patient information should not be discussed in public areas," mentioned in Chapter 2, is important to embrace.

Cell phones and other communication

The healthcare practitioner's office has numerous opportunities for unwanted sound to disturb patients (and staff): patients' cell phones, office telephones, office equipment, and staff talking to each other. Practitioners often post a notice in the reception area indicating that cell phone use is either prohibited or discouraged; with the popularity of texting, the problem of unwanted conversations may diminish. To post a cell phone policy, you need a notice board, which could be mounted on a wall in the reception area.

In the reception area, one recommendation is to have a separate telephone room where staff place calls for patient appointment reminders and schedule follow-up tests; yet such tests are often scheduled as the patient leaves the office, typically overlapping with the reception area. As such, these conversations are often audible (or could be). For such reasons, the use of a music system in the waiting room (discussed in Chapter 4) may help mask conversation.

To reduce sound, systems to signal staff and physicians about a needed call can be handled through a panel of lights in the exam room and consultation rooms, a recommendation made by Malkin.[41] Another system is an intercom, although this can typically be heard by unintended others if it connects to the staff work area. Malkin also recommends an auditory signal system, using an annunciator panel, where different tones can be associated with a different physician and a different action (e.g., Dr. Smith needs an assistant to do an EKG).

Summary of design considerations

In reducing unwanted sound, two themes emerge in the literature: adjacencies and materials. Spatially, locating functions likely to produce noise (such as office machines) in areas away from patients (both in waiting and in clinical settings) can reduce unwanted sound. Materials that are sound absorbing also address the problem and increase speech intelligibility while simultaneously decreasing violations of speech privacy.

The electronic office and doctor-patient communication (DPC)

The federal government requires EMRs to be phased in by 2015, after which those who cannot demonstrate "meaningful use" of such EMR systems will face penalties in the form of deductions in Medicare reimbursement rates. EMRs are here to stay. Eventually EMRs may lead to greater efficiencies in medical offices, but training in the use of the systems is involved. Whatever system is selected (e-scribe, tablet pc, desktop pc, a combination, speech recognition),[42] the essential goal should be direct communication with the patient; that is, establishing eye contact, listening, communicating empathy, responding to questions. If the technology interferes with these fundamental processes, outcomes for patients may be negatively affected.

When practitioners meet with patients, those practitioners who are still developing expertise with EMR systems may spend time looking at the screen and not the patient. Research on how electronic technology impacts the doctor-patient relationship is beginning to accumulate. A review of research by Shachak and Reis revealed both positive and negative effects of EMRs on DPC. Use of EMRs can facilitate the exchange of information about biomedical issues; at the same time, the patient-centeredness of the interaction can decrease. When physicians spent as much as 25 percent of the time in the consultation gazing at the screen, for example, and similarly were typing as much as 24 percent of the time (described as heavy keyboarding), the quality of the communication decreased and rapport was often lost. The more time spent in gazing at the screen, the lower the involvement of the physician in asking questions of the patient; consequently emotional responsiveness also dropped.[43]

Medical students are the practitioners of tomorrow; with 3rd year medical students, a sizable percentage of them (over 60 percent) were satisfied with the DPC, but almost 50 percent acknowledged they spent less time looking at the patient when the EMR was used compared to traditional paper records. Moreover, only 21 percent of these 3rd year students strongly agreed/agreed with the statement, "My patients liked that I was using an EHR."[44] Skill in using technology and simultaneously developing an interpersonal bond with patients is challenging and points to possible negative effects of multitasking. Researchers suggest that physicians using EMRs with patients separate the tasks;[45] that is, there is a time for talking and a time for typing. In this way, the patient-centered quality of the interaction can be preserved.

One early objection to reading from a screen was a drop in comprehension; however, recent evidence suggests that the reading comprehension of medical professionals is comparable whether reading on a screen or from a paper copy. That performance notwithstanding, in a study of over 100 medical professionals, 90 percent preferred reading on paper to electronic screens;[46] this finding was not related to the practitioner's age, level of expertise, or domain of knowledge. The medical professionals in this study also commented on the haptic qualities paper possesses; they like the way paper feels in their hands.

Monitor position

One of the important aspects of DPC is where the computer monitor is positioned,[47] which in turn affects how it can be used. In new office construction, suites "are prewired for computers with extra wall plugs, flat-panel monitors in exam rooms and a small locked room for the computer server."[48] But where will the technology be placed? Can it be wall-mounted to swivel out and back into place, flush with the wall? Might it offer more flexibility on a movable cart or table, as shown in Figure 3.10? It is likely that the flexibility provided by transportable computer equipment will be seen as a major advantage to practitioners given the rate with which such technology changes.

From the standpoint of design, a number of aspects can facilitate DPC when a computer and monitor are involved. Fixed-position screens may interfere with the physician's ability to directly face the patient. For that reason, movable monitors on adjustable arms, which allow the doctor to position the monitor to share information with the patient, are useful. In addition, when there are multiple locations in the office where EMRs can be viewed, Shachak and Reis[49] suggest there is more choice about when to access these records. Technology in the office suite is a moving target; in all likelihood miniaturization of such equipment will continue. One of the best questions practitioners and designers can continue to ask is "What if…?" and imagine the planning needed for a range of possibilities, from complete portability to unmovable fixtures.

Researchers point out that computer placement is critical to the quality of the communication between doctors and their patients; for that reason, such considerations are important as the

Consultation and Examination Spaces 91

space is planned, yet the role of the physical environment in DPC is not necessarily considered.[50] These concerns may diminish when practitioners use wireless handheld devices (e.g., computer tablets), but a larger mounted screen may be necessary for both practitioner and patient to easily view the information.

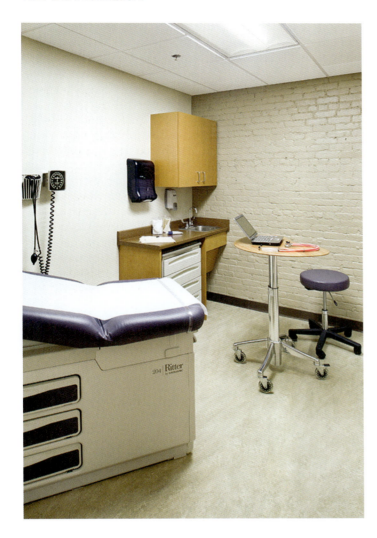

Figure 3.10: *Movable table and drawers (underneath the wall cabinetry) support technology and clinical functions.*
Location: Thundermist Health Center, West Warwick, Rhode Island.
Architect: Vision 3 Architects.
Photo credit: Aaron Usher III Photography

Illumination: Properties of lighting and dynamic lighting systems

The difference between appropriate lighting levels in the exam and consultation spaces points to an important principle: one size doesn't fit all. A single lighting level will not work across situations. For that reason, having 1) more than one source of lighting, and 2) adjustable lighting is important to provide more control for both patients and staff. As but one example of the facilitative effect of lighting, an interviewer in a therapy setting was evaluated in four different conditions (varying two levels of lighting and two of decoration). Dimmer lighting was associated with higher pleasantness-calmness scores than the bright lighting condition. The dim lighting condition also had an impact on disclosure, increasing the amount of time the interviewee spent talking.[51]

This recommendation of dim lighting may generalize beyond therapy settings to some medical contexts. Dimmer lighting would be appropriate in a consultation room but not an exam room. The effect of lighting should be considered as practitioners strive to make the environment of consultation one that encourages dialogue and disclosure, whatever the medical condition. Readers desiring more detail about the kind of cues that lighting provides are directed to Flynn's 1992 book on architectural interiors,[52] which addresses lighting cue theory.

In the context of the healthcare office, a number of different functions require different illumination. Lighting levels have to be higher where people are working on computer screens, such as the administrative area; lighting levels have to be bright enough in hallways where patients walk to lower the risk of falling. Exterior lighting, for example on pathways and in the parking lot, also has to be sufficient to guide movement, especially in the late afternoon when sunlight may not be sufficient. In general, brighter lighting is needed in procedure areas, whereas dimmer lighting is appropriate in consultation and waiting areas. Arneill and Frasca-Beaulieu not only see lighting as a way to provide a comfortable environment but also as one that allows the patient to exert some control – for example, by adjusting blinds or dimmers. In waiting areas, by combining "different types of lighting, such as recessed fluorescent downlighting for general illumination, accent wallwashers to highlight artwork, and floor and table lamps for reading, designers can create a residential atmosphere that feels more comfortable, supportive, and nurturing,"[53] as illustrated in Figure 3.11.

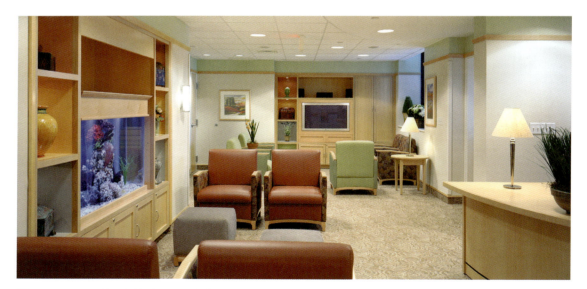

Figure 3.11: *Residential lighting, soft furniture, and positive distractions provide a patient-centered atmosphere.*
Location: Griffin Hospital, Inpatient Psychiatric Unit, Derby, Connecticut.
Architect: The S/L/A/M Collaborative.
Photo credit: Woodruff/Brown Architectural Photography

Consultation and Examination Spaces

A list of recommendations for improving lighting in healthcare environments comes form Benya.[54] Among these recommendations are reducing glare, increasing daylight, using softer and less institutional lighting, and consideration of the color temperatures of light (warm, cool, or in the middle). Lamps that range in the zone between warm to cool, in the neighborhood of 3500 kelvins, are common.[55]

Essentially, he says, eliminate the use of fluorescent lighting in public and patient areas and focus on lighting with a residential flavor. Such fixtures, he says, would be floor and table lamps, lamps that have swing-arms, and track lighting. Consistent with our theme of control, he notes that dimmers offer flexibility. Relative to the costs of other types of architectural improvements, lighting has an effect "far greater in both aesthetic and psychological value."[56] Further, as he points out, lighting enhances patient safety through adequately illuminating indoor corridors (paths) and emergency egresses. Lighting also provides security around the building.

Natural light

Where possible, natural lighting should be emphasized. The fact that the lab and emergency department waiting area in Figure 3.12 is next to an entrance with natural light makes spending time in this small space more positive.

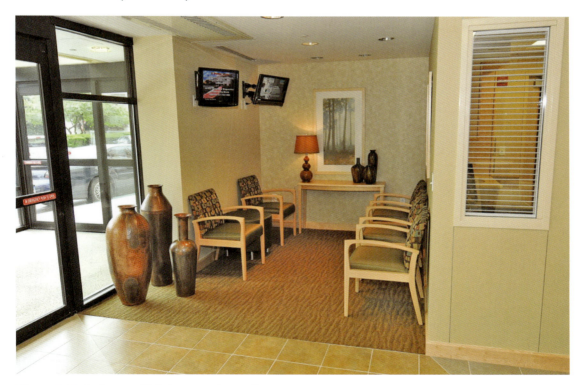

Figure 3.12: A vista outside helps expand a small space.
Location: Griffin Hospital, Emergency Department, Derby, Connecticut.
Architect: The S/L/A/M Collaborative.
Photo credit: The S/L/A/M Collaborative

The recommendation to use natural light cannot always be followed – for example, when medical offices are located adjacent to the interior corridors in office buildings – but the amount of natural light available in the office suite should be a consideration as practitioners choose among sites to rent or purchase. Figure 3.13, from the Thundermist Health Center, shows how clerestory lighting can be used to help illuminate interior corridors. Commonly known as the Cotton Shed, this health facility was created out of a cotton fabric storage facility, situated across the street from the mill itself, which functioned in the Civil War era. With limited possibilities for natural light in the stone building, the use of these clerestory windows contributes to the success of the project.

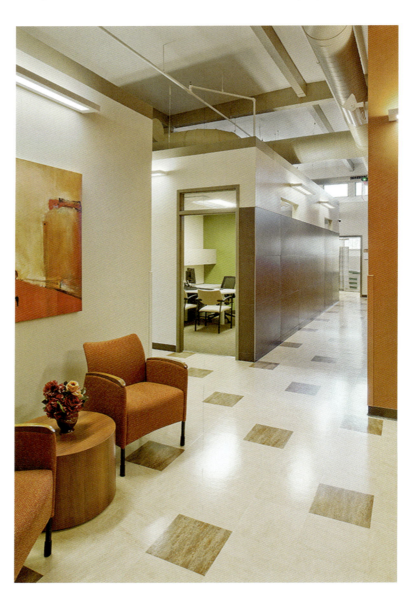

Figure 3.13: *Use of clerestory windows provides natural light to interior corridors.*
Location: Thundermist Health Center, West Warwick, Rhode Island.
Architect: Vision 3 Architects.
Photo credit: Aaron Usher III Photography

In inpatient rooms, morning light is more beneficial than afternoon light, in terms of reducing average length of stay. Practitioners selecting office sites should consider the location of the office suite vis-à-vis the site to see which spaces would receive morning or afternoon light.[57] Skylights are another consideration. High levels of illumination, especially in the morning, have been associated with positive outcomes.[58]

Dynamic lighting

Recently, systems have been introduced that can vary the levels of interior lighting over the course of the day. These systems, called dynamic lighting, can be adjusted to vary the level of light and the color temperature produced.[59] Practitioners may want more light in the morning and after lunch (when levels of alertness drop) and may want to soften the light for patients (not necessarily for staff) at other times of the day – for example, in the later afternoon. Definitive effects of dynamic lighting are not established, but there is some evidence that mood can be enhanced using it, judging by self-report indicators. At the very least, the opportunity for variability offers one more aspect of control in the environment even if staff members (not patients) control the system.

Effects of lighting on staff

In addition to the effects of light on vision (such as the amount of light necessary for reading), light has the potential to affect well-being and performance. We tend to emphasize the effects of lighting for patients, but such effects are important for staff as well. Research suggests that light can be used to combat fatigue and loss of vitality; it also demonstrates the need to have variable control of lighting to change illumination as the task or desired outcomes demand.[60] This research points to the importance of being able to control task lighting; when you are tired, especially at the end of the day, being able to turn up the lighting may help maintain alertness. In addition, when staff work areas have access to natural light, even rather modestly furnished spaces are more pleasant.

Personalization in the office suite

For physicians, there may be advantages to the display of professional credentials, art objects, and mementos, as long as the display is organized. In a primary territory like a personal office, physicians have control over personal objects and how many they display. In shared spaces like the reception area and front office, some limit is encouraged to promote a professional look.[61] Shared space can easily become cluttered.

There is considerable research about the role of personalization in the office environment. Offices can be both functional and ceremonial.[62] Americans personalize their offices, and estimates are that upwards of 70 percent do so; those of higher status are more likely to make themselves known through displays.[63] Research on psychotherapists suggests displaying diplomas and certifications is important.[64] If the private office is used as a consultation space, patients will look for evidence that the doctor is qualified. This information is available on the Internet, but seeing it reinforces that knowledge.

Research on psychotherapists' offices suggests that orderliness is valued; for that reason, the physician's office should provide options for storage, including bookshelves and containers for pharmaceutical samples. Unless there is sufficient storage, starter samples provided by pharmaceutical sales representatives may pile up and create clutter in the office.

The social psychologist Sam Gosling describes how office displays communicate clues to personality. Using a personality inventory that targets five traits, known as the Big 5 (openness to experience, conscientiousness, extroversion, agreeableness, neuroticism), research showed people make inferences about a room's occupant from the artifacts in the room. In this research, conscientiousness was negatively related to room clutter, which suggests that people associate neat and tidy spaces with individuals who are high on conscientiousness. In Gosling's research, the variables "good use of space," "clean," and "organized," were positively correlated with judgments of conscientiousness; "cluttered" was negatively correlated with judgments of conscientiousness. Other correlations with conscientiousness point to the schema one might have of a doctor's office. Succinctly, this research describes the physical environment of a conscientious person (someone who might be a doctor) as roomy, expensive, in good condition, more empty than full, comfortable, inviting, and formal.[65] The private office in Figure 3.14 is a highly personalized and welcoming space; the presence of diplomas produces a sufficiently formal impression.

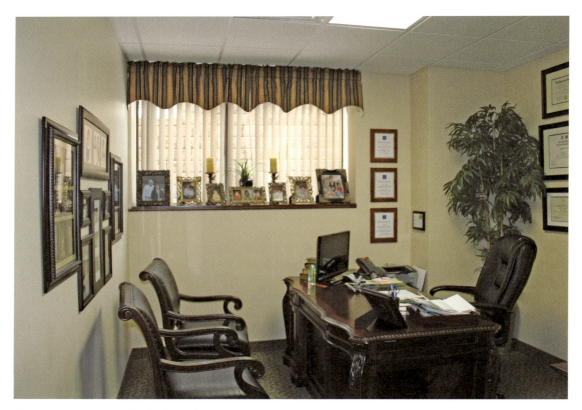

Figure 3.14: *A personalized office welcomes patients.*
Location: *Office of Neeraj Kohli, MD MBA, Wellesley, Massachusetts.*

The psychotherapist's office: Continuous consultation and examination

The psychotherapy office provides the unique case in which every session simultaneously includes both exam and consultation in the same room; the talking often is the cure. In a solo practice, which may be more common in psychotherapy than in other aspects of healthcare, the psychotherapist's office is typically the practitioner's own office as well as the space in which psychotherapy is conducted. Other aspects of the nature of the profession are also reflected in its space and its layout. These include special pressures to safeguard patients' privacy, reflected in the flow of people through the office and the location of the restroom.

Often psychotherapy sessions involve considerable emotion on the part of the client; people may be emotionally distraught when they leave. The client needs a "way out" that helps to save face. In other words, the layout of the office is particularly important in providing a means of egress that involves little (ideally no) contact with others.

The spatial layout

In psychotherapy, in particular, there is pressure to safeguard the patient's privacy as stigma is still attached to seeing a therapist; even within the profession itself, negative attitudes remain.[66] In a group practice, there is typically a waiting room with a receptionist's window. At check in, the receptionist collects fees, which may involve co-payments for insurance or the full amount of the session if insurance is not accepted. Often, a doorway from the waiting area leads to a corridor off of which therapists' offices are located. At the conclusion of sessions, practitioners themselves schedule clients' next appointments, eliminating a second interaction with the receptionist. The interior corridor extending down the row of therapists' offices can exit directly into the building hallway. In this manner, undesirable contact with others is reduced. The client who is distraught need not face a waiting room full of yet-to-be-seen clients.

The view

Having a view, preferably to nature, is important for any practitioner, but it is particularly relevant in the psychotherapy office where, session after session, the client and practitioner do "the work" of therapy. Psychotherapy is one of the professions in which delivering counseling in an office is likely to remain viable, even as the availability and use of teletherapies grow. Having a vista to nature, and ideally two walls of windows (e.g., in a corner office), creates a supportive visual environment for therapy.

Design issues in telemedicine and teletherapy

Telemedicine, the approach to medicine (diagnosis, treatment) via remote communication, is being adopted by psychotherapists. In psychotherapy, the core of the treatment involves communication. With the availability of such technologies as Skype, the exchanges in psychotherapy can be managed this way, at least in some cases. What does this have to do with the physical environment? HIPAA plays a central role in the practice management of any kind of medicine, and that is true with telemedicine and teletherapy. In addition to the layers of security required in telemedicine, the position of the computer in the office plays a role. Patients want to see that the door to the physician's or psychotherapist's office is closed; with the practitioner's back to the door, patients can observe whether the door opens at any time during the session. In an article discussing online therapy, a therapist was quoted to say that he wears a headset to make sure clients appreciate the safeguard for privacy being taken.[67]

In terms of design, lighting was mentioned as a consideration, as it can distort the way the practitioner looks; for that reason it was recommended that the practitioner try out how he or she looks to a potential client by interfacing with other clinicians online. The limited evaluation research on the topic indicates positive results, reviewed in an article by Simpson.[68] She points out that some patients may experience a greater sense of control in their own environment using their own technological equipment; for others who have less comfort with technology, this approach may cause anxiety.

Restrooms: Group and individual practice

Giving a urine sample during an annual exam in a physician's office is routine. For a psychotherapy visit in the office of a solo practitioner, use of the restroom within the psychotherapist's suite may raise boundary and privacy issues for the client. A goal of psychotherapy is a kind of emotional transparency, not a physical one.

A restroom is nevertheless needed for the practitioner and client (if he/she chooses to use it) within the office, but having a restroom available to clients outside the office is desirable as well. This arrangement gives the client choice, which is an important consideration and one of the central design principles in this book. One client used a restroom at a gasoline station within a quarter mile of the practitioner's office rather than within the practitioner's suite. There was no restroom available in the semi-public space of the office building. A solution, both for group and solo practice, is the provision of restrooms on each floor of an office building in which the psychotherapy practice is located. In this way, clients have a choice to use the restroom in the office suite or not. Using the restroom outside of the suite typically provides clients with a greater degree of privacy and control than is true of a restroom within the suite.

Security considerations: The role of design

Psychotherapists may deal with patients with a propensity for violence. The office layout may provide some degree of safety in terms of a hierarchy of spaces. In group practice, the semi-public waiting area is often separated from a corridor of private therapy offices by a door that can be locked to prevent access to these offices. In addition, in a group practice, a door exiting to the public hallway from the interior corridor lining the row of therapists' offices is locked from the hallway side to prevent access to the corridor from the public hallway. These lockable doors serve a gatekeeper function.

The physical environment is one of a number of variables to be assessed when dealing with the potential of client violence. Other variables include clinical risk markers, personality features and personality disorders, and substance abuse backgrounds. Having a space between the client and the therapist (e.g., a coffee table between them) is desirable. Newhill also advises having solid furniture that is difficult to move or throw; removing heavy objects (e.g., statues) that might be used as projectiles; and sitting between the client and the door. Therapists, she notes, should have a means to signal for help that is prearranged. This signal might be an emergency call button on a phone, for example.[69]

How furnishings and décor influence clients' judgments of the therapist

A number of recent studies[70] point to the effect of furnishings and décor on judgments of the practitioner, including the quality of care to be delivered and the comfort the client feels in the setting. In evaluating respondents' attitudes toward a therapist whose office was viewed, researchers manipulated the number of credentials (none, two, four, or nine) and family photographs (none or two) on display.[71] Judgments of the therapist's qualifications, friendliness, and energy were impacted by the number of diplomas and credentials displayed, but not by the presence or absence of family photographs. More positive views of the therapist's qualifications occurred with four credentials displayed than with fewer than that, but no advantage emerged with nine credentials. For the therapist's energy or dynamism, displaying nine credentials had the greatest impact. The findings indicated no difference by experience in therapy or not, suggesting these results might generalize across levels of experience and perhaps across office types. With the number of credentials displayed in the office, Figure 3.14 shows an office likely to impress patients.

In the study, participants were asked to explain their ratings, which yielded qualitative comments. Beyond responses dealing specifically with the diplomas and photographs, 60 percent of the participants pointed out something negative about the environment, which admittedly was somewhat bland. These comments related to the lack of personalization, art, and color; the overall blandness and starkness of the office; the uncomfortable-looking furnishings; and the lack of plants. This study used photographs taken in a practicing therapist's office, suggesting that practitioners might benefit from advice about their office décor.

In related research, the images of 30 psychotherapists' offices, taken by the photographer Saul Robbins, led to a series of studies examining the appearance of the office on judgments of the therapist. The photographs were taken in Manhattan; each photograph showed the view of the therapist's chair in the office, taken from the vantage point a client would have.[72] In three studies,[73] [74] [75] the core results revealed a pattern. Judgments of the therapist improved as the orderliness and softness/personalization of the office increased.

Orderliness in the office is an issue that healthcare professionals, whatever their specialty, may want to consider. Similarly, softness and personalization are valuable tools to create a comfortable environment for the client. Considering how comfortable the chairs are to sit in and what there is to look at (art, books, color, vistas out a window) can benefit both the patient and practitioner. These findings regarding softness/personalization suggest the importance of furnishings reflecting a residential tone.

Consultation and exam spaces: A century ago

Physicians practicing in the early 1900s faced decisions about how many rooms their office would have. Like the admonitions that appeared from Cathell about office location (shared in Chapter 1), periodicals such as *The Office Practitioner* and manuals of the day emphasized putting some effort into securing a sufficient number of rooms and furnishing them appropriately. As Mathews warns, "Don't be persuaded, or persuade yourself, that any 'old thing' will do, for it will not."[76] A minimum of two rooms seemed to be the standard,[77] with one used as a general office or reception room, sometimes called a coating room, the other as a formal examination/treatment room. This second (examination) room provided privacy, but doctors were advised to take special precautions when performing a gynecological examination there. In these instances, an assistant or a patient's friend was to be present;[78] practitioners today follow the same practice of having an assistant present for pelvic exams. The room was to be well lighted, and an office with windows on two walls was preferable,[79] foreshadowing the importance of having natural light in medical facilities today.

In the early office, the exam room could also be used as an operating room – a vast improvement to surgery in the patient's home. One story about my paternal grandfather describes him amputating a patient's leg on the patient's kitchen table. "Before he came to Clarksburg, Dr. Sloan had assisted his father in 'kitchen table' surgery in the city of Marietta, Ohio. On the day of the scheduled surgery the two doctors, before they left their office, sterilized the instruments they would use and carried the instruments with them in a covered container."[80] My grandfather was still performing such amputations on patients' kitchen tables (with ether administered) in 1910.[81]

An article in *The Office Practitioner* in 1905[82] argues that attention to the office setting could help build a successful practice. The author commented on the disorder and dirt (including cobwebs hanging from the ceiling) he found in a physician's office and that same physician's bewilderment about how few patients he saw in his small practice. The author makes the direct association between the impression created by the office and income (dollars).

Despite this advice, some practitioners overlooked the impact of the physical environment. The spittoon was ever present as tobacco chewing was common, and decorative features such as wallpaper, rug, and sofa, if present, were likely to be worn and faded; newspapers and magazines, if available, were likely to be old.[83] We may not see spittoons in the office today, but the research on psychotherapists' offices suggests practitioners might benefit from guidance regarding office ambiance.

Who decorates? The silent partner

A reference to "the little woman" in advice manuals of the time underscores a theme prevalent in much of the literature about medicine in the late nineteenth and early twentieth century. The wife, sometimes referred to as the silent partner, was an important asset. The wife helped in decorating, cleaning, and otherwise having insight into the finer things in life. She could be counted on to oversee the decoration of the office. The wife was responsible for providing the finishing touches, the pattern of the wallpaper, a rug, decorations for the mantelpiece, and pictures, given what Mathews' 1905 book describes as her "deft fingers and quick perception."[84] The display of flowers, either cut or growing, reflected a cultured taste; the office was to be "fresh, neat, clean, and scientific."[85]

Furnishings in the office were one indication of the physician's cultivation. According to *The Office Practitioner*, the physician needed durable furniture, not easily marred, consisting of a desk, chairs, and bookshelves. A desk with pigeonholes was desirable (to organize notes and

Consultation and Examination Spaces 101

bills). An examination table, cabinet for instruments, shelves for medicines, mortar and pestle, and apothecary scale were required. Chairs (one or two) were needed, with rockers recommended for female patients. An easy chair for the physician permitted comfort in reading when time permitted. The bookcase was important to reflect positively on the physician, and a revolving bookstand for reference books was recommended.[86]

In addition to equipment and furniture in the office, physicians also needed objects related to hygiene (slop jar, washstand, pitcher, towels, toilet articles). Physicians were advised to keep these articles for hygiene out of sight, foreshadowing hospital practice in the twenty-first century in which cabinets, screens, and drawers in patients' rooms hide soiled linen, trash, and medical debris. Then, as now, patients did not like to be reminded of the remnants of any medical procedure and are bothered by clutter and disorder in the medical setting. There is increased emphasis on the use of screening through cabinetry to address this issue of clutter and views of equipment in medical offices (see Figure 3.15). Even simple bifold doors can be used in this regard (see Figure 3.16).

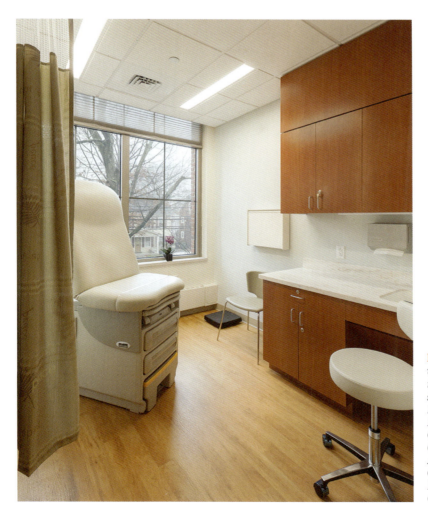

Figure 3.15: *The cabinets' warm wood tones soften the room and provide elegant storage and screening. Location: Greenwich Hospital, Bendheim Cancer Center, Greenwich, Connecticut. Architect: The S/L/A/M Collaborative. Photo credit: John Giammatteo*

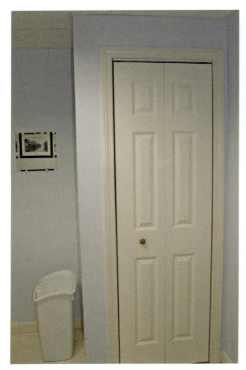 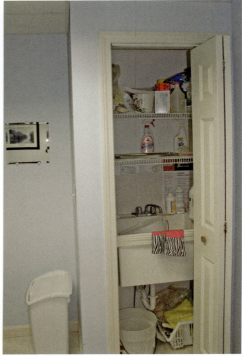

Figure 3.16: *Simple bifold doors screen a sink and cleaners.*
Location: Office of Timothy Barczak, MD, New London, Connecticut.

Further Reading

Agency for Healthcare Research and Quality. *Making Health Care Safer: A Critical Analysis of Patient Safety Practices.* Rockville, MD: AHRQ, 2001.
Benya, James R. "Lighting for Healing." *Journal of Health Care Interior Design* 1, (1989): 55–58.
Cahnman, Sheila F. "Outpatient Options: A Look at the Changing Ambulatory Care Facility." *Health Facilities Management.* June, 2011. http://www.hfmmagazine.com/hfmmagazine/jsp/articledisplay.jsp?dcrpath=HFMMAGAZINE/Article/data/06JUN2011/0611HFM_FEA_AD&domain=HFMMAGAZINE
Casciato, Daniel. "Soundproofing Your Office." *Medical Office Today.* August 17, 2010. http://www.medicalofficetoday.com/article/soundproofing-your-office.aspx
Frampton, Susan B., Laura Gilpin, and Patrick A. Charmel. *Putting Patients First: Designing and Practicing Patient-Centered Care.* San Francisco, CA: Jossey-Bass, 2003.
Flynn, John E. *Architectural Interior Systems: Lighting, Acoustics, and Air Conditioning,* 3rd ed. New York: Van Nostrand Reinhold, 1992.
Green Guide for Health Care™. *Acoustic Environment Technical Brief.* Green Guide for Health Care™. Version 2.2, 2007. http://www.gghc.org/documents/TechBriefs/GGHC_TechBrief_Acoustic-Environment.pdf
Gulwadi, Gowri Betrabet, Anjali Joseph, and Amy Beth Keller. "Exploring the Impact of the Physical Environment on Patient Outcomes in Ambulatory Care Settings." *Health Environments Research & Design Journal* 2(2), (2009): 21–41. http://www.herdjournal.com/article/exploring-impact-physical-environment-patient-outcomes-ambulatory-care-settings

HermanMiller Healthcare. "Sound Practices: Noise Control in the Healthcare Environment. Research Summary" HermanMiller Healthcare. Research Summary, 2006. http://www.hermanmiller.com/content/hermanmiller/english/research/research-summaries/sound-practices-noise-control-in-the-healthcare-environment.html

Joseph, Anjali, and Roger Ulrich. "Sound Control for Improved Outcomes in Healthcare Settings." Issue Paper 4. The Center for Health Design. January, 2007. http://www.healthdesign.org/sites/default/files/Sound%20Control.pdf

McColl, Shelley L., and Jennifer A. Veitch. "Full-spectrum Fluorescent Lighting: A Review of Its Effects on Physiology and Health." *Psychological Medicine* 31(6), (2001): 949–964. doi:10.1017/S003329170105425

Nasar, Jack L. and Ann Sloan Devlin. "Impressions of Psychotherapists' Offices." *Journal of Counseling Psychology* 58(3), (2011): 310–320. doi:10.1037/a00238872011

Shachak, Aviv, and Shmuel Reis. "The Impact of Electronic Medical Records on Patient-Doctor Communication During Consultation: A Narrative Literature Review." *Journal of Evaluation in Clinical Practice* 15(4), (2009): 641–649. doi:10.1111/j.1365-2753.2008.01065.x

Veitch, Jennifer A., and McColl, Shelley L. "A Critical Examination of Perceptual Cognitive Effects Attributed to Full-Spectrum Fluorescent Lighting." *Ergonomics* 44(3), (2001): 255–279, 255. doi:10.1080/00140130010002008

Weidman, Ted. "Psychologist Office Sound Problem." Acoustical Surfaces-Soundproofing Blog. July 24, 2008. http://www.acousticalsurfaces.com/blog/soundproofing/psychologist-office-sound-problem/

The Ambient Environment:
Changing the "Sick People's" Atmosphere

4

Overview: The waiting room should "lose its 'sick people's' atmosphere"

When cancer patients were asked how waiting rooms could be improved, they said the facility should "lose its 'sick people's atmosphere.'"[1] People don't want to be reminded of illness; physicians and designers must consider how an environment can instead communicate wellness. Many of these aspects can be communicated to our senses, the focus of this chapter.

During a visit to a healthcare provider, aspects of the environment will impinge on visual, auditory, olfactory, and tactile senses and will also affect thermal comfort. "In progressing from parking to entry to lobby and then entering into the health facility, what one sees, hears, smells, touches, and tastes is vital to a holistic, thoughtful, patient-centered environment."[2] This statement was made in reference to Planetree facilities but is applicable to healthcare facilities more generally.

Ambient characteristics: Control, positive distraction, and personalization

The ambient environment refers to the environment that surrounds us, in particular to air quality and sound, but more broadly to the sense of the environment – to sights, sounds, smells, and touch. When people enter a nursing home, a positive response might be "This place doesn't 'smell,'" reflecting their association between nursing homes and odors like stale urine or air freshener to cover mustiness. Our schemas thus include the sensory environment. Patients control little of what happens to them in the medical arena; the ambient characteristics of the environment offer the opportunity to redress that imbalance, whether it is adjusting the lighting level in the waiting room or selecting a current magazine to read.

In other instances the environment offers comfort and reassurance – for example, to drink a beverage in the waiting room or feel the softness of a chair cushion. Fabric-covered seating, nature photographs on the walls, and live potted plants have been associated with positive mood and high levels of satisfaction among patients in a waiting area.[3] In this research, the authors note a positive response can emerge without a large outlay of capital. The interventions were not structural but instead involved changes in a number of design features, from lighting to furnishings and color. Similar effects have been demonstrated in intervention research in the waiting area of a dental practice.[4]

Giving patients control and permission

Patients may need help asserting control over the environment. They may need both education and permission. For example, patients differ in their degree of sophistication with regard to technology. They may need instruction to use whatever technology is provided. Receptionists could demonstrate the use of the equipment (e.g., a check-in kiosk), or distribute a step-by-step handout when patients check in.

A second important aspect is permission. When patients enter a healthcare facility, their schema is one of relinquishing control. This schema needs modification. Patients need to know they may turn on or adjust the lighting level of lamps. It is important for healthcare providers to give patients permission to exert some control over the environment.

The senses: Visual stimulation and positive distraction

Humans are often described as visual animals; the visual system occupies a substantial amount of the cerebral cortex – more than the area devoted to the other senses.[5] Relevant to the practitioner's office, what opportunities for positive visual distraction exist in each space? Positive distractions are aspects of the environment that divert the patient's attention from negative aspects of the visit (e.g., an impending inoculation) to positive aspects of the environment (e.g., a view to nature).

The 180-degree principle

Consider what could be called the 180-degree principle. Layout and placement need to reinforce customary behavior, which puts an emphasis on what is in front and back of us (as we move into and out of the office). What is noticed is directly in front of the patient, with a viewing angle probably not more than 20 degrees to the left and to the right unless the head is moved.[6] Further, as people age, their range of motion becomes limited; they are less likely to turn their heads. In other words, the emphasis throughout the suite needs to be on what is seen coming and going. Henderson suggests that knowledge of schemas will direct where people look in a given scene; they look where they expect relevant objects to be and apprehend the gist of the scene very rapidly – typically within the length of a single fixation, which may last less than half a second.[7]

Related to wayfinding, people tend to look toward landmarks at the end of hallways or T-junctions;[8] that is, to look where they are going. A view at the end of a corridor, as seen in Figure 4.01, can help them with orientation.

The height of any object displayed on the wall is also relevant. ADA standards dictate that signage be posted 60 inches above the floor to the finish line of the sign.[9] Signs or artwork hung above that level are typically outside of where we normally look because we do not expect objects to be posted any higher.

I sat for what was at least the thirtieth time in my practitioner's personal office on a recent visit. Entering this office used for consultation, which the practitioner keeps dimly lighted (and appropriately so, in my view), I took my seat directly across the desk from him, as I always do. Given

The Ambient Environment

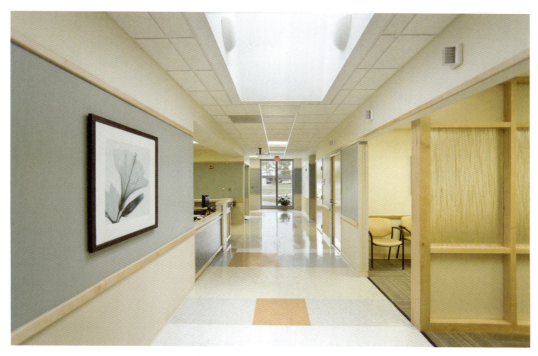

Figure 4.01: *Vista provides light and a wayfinding cue.*
Location: Onslow Hospital, Radiation Oncology Center, Jacksonville, North Carolina.
Architect: The S/L/A/M Collaborative.
Photo credit: John Giammatteo

this book project, I also turned my head to look at the wall to my immediate left. In over 30 visits to this office, I had never looked to the left because the visitor/patient chair is placed very close to the wall. There on the wall were ten diplomas and certificates. In 30 visits I had never "noticed" them because my attention was directly forward, looking at the practitioner.

Positive distraction: The debate surrounding television

The advantages and disadvantages of television, specifically in the waiting room, need to be carefully weighed; within the framework of control, what might be considered an asset (i.e., positive distraction) may become a liability. Research suggests as much. Stress levels in patients waiting to donate blood at a blood bank were actually higher when the television was turned on than off. This was a large study, with almost 900 participants, and a field experiment, not a simulation. These blood donors were distributed across a variety of visual conditions displayed on a monitor; these conditions represented nature, the built environment, network daytime programming (no news), and a blank monitor. The waiting room was described as "comfortable, attractive, non-institutional with overstuffed chairs, sofas, coffee tables with magazines, and carpeting."[10] Findings reflected positive effects for nature, but more noteworthy was that having television turned off was preferable, at least with regard to the physiological measures, to having it turned on. The authors comment, "healthcare administrators and designers should think twice before exposing stressed consumers to uncontrollable daytime television."[11]

Similarly, in describing the comforting aspects of Planetree facilities, Arneill and Frasca-Beaulieu recommend against a television in waiting areas;[12] as do Mazer and Smith: "The television dominates any environment in which it is running. If it is not appropriately part of the healing environment, then it is violating it."[13] When people are kept waiting, the uncontrollability of the television viewing situation is likely to contribute to stress.[14] Further, a number of authors worry about television news that includes violence. Close-captioning or use of headphones (hygienic) borrowed from the reception desk might help increase patients' sense of control.[15] Any number of posts on healthcare websites show that the issue of television is problematic.[16]

Why television is viewed as a positive distraction

Positive distraction is necessary because of the length of time spent in the waiting room. As mentioned earlier in this book, during the renovation of the waiting area for adults in the Emergency Department at Yale-New Haven Hospital, administrators removed the television precisely because they thought it signaled "a long wait" to patients, a message they did not want to send.

The relationship between waiting time and satisfaction with service is well established; but the attractiveness of the waiting room environment may enhance mood, and the presence of television may play a role once boredom sets in, argue Pruyn and Smidts.[17] The authors suggest that after

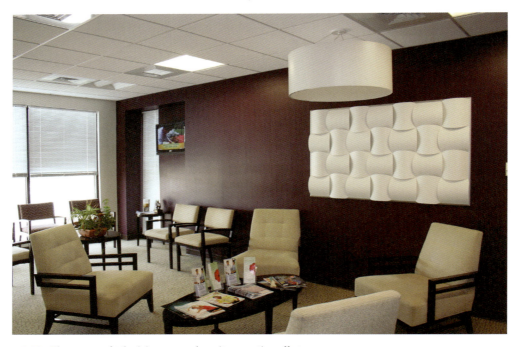

Figure 4.02: *Placement of television can reduce its negative effects.*
Location: Women & Infants Center for Reproduction and Infertility, Providence, Rhode Island.

The Ambient Environment

self-paced distractions (like reading magazines) have been exhausted, people have no option but to turn to whatever stimulation remains: television. If you want patients to perceive that less time has passed, they suggest showing programs that last longer and depict fewer topics. In their research, segmentation (i.e., more clips) increased the perception that more time had passed. In fairness to television, some research shows that patients recommend television, as was the case in a large study in Taiwan (over 140,000 patients) in 17 different outpatient clinics. Patients recommended more reading materials, and a third wanted television installed on the wall.[18] In the absence of knowing what visual alternatives there might be, people may recommend television.

When the clinical staff decides in favor of television, there are ways to make it less prominent. Some designers minimize the impact of television through seating zones in the waiting area. In the photograph in Figure 4.02, designers placed the television at one end of the waiting area, recessed into a niche, to avoid having the television dominate the space.

Alternatives to television

The notion of nature that is simulated, sometimes called mediated nature, defined as "natural images or figures translated into another medium,"[19] may be a good alternative to daytime programmed television, according to Mazer. She suggests such mediated nature could be found in film documentaries, photographs, the Discovery Channel, specials from National Geographic, and NOVA, among other possibilities. An audio tape of soothing music, specifically designed for healthcare environments (see section on music in this chapter), can accompany the visual images, or those images can be used by themselves. A loop of soothing music and associated nature photographs, available on the CARE Channel (Continuous Ambient Relaxation Environment), has been suggested as an appropriate alternative to reduce stress.[20] An example of nature images on a loop is seen in Figure 4.03, in the waiting room of a small practice.

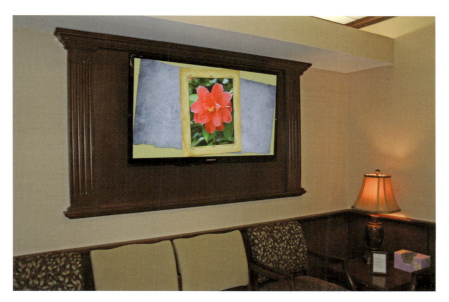

Figure 4.03: *A loop of nature images displayed on a waiting room monitor. Location: Office of Neeraj Kohli, MD MBA, Wellesley, Massachusetts.*

Nature images are provided by a number of firms (e.g., American Art Resources, Art Research Institute, Healing HealthCare Systems®).

How else might patients be distracted in the waiting room? Caroline Leemis suggests a three-pronged attack: displaying artwork, clustering seating, and offering technology. Her ideas for artwork include rotating gallery-like displays using art produced by artisans in the local community, pointing out that patients will see something new on each visit. With regard to technology, she suggests providing computers at small stations (see Figure 2.21). For patients who bring their technology with them, she endorses wireless networks.[21]

Another possibility is an aquarium,[22] used as an alternative to television at the Smilow Cancer Hospital in Connecticut. A monitor could also show aquatic images, as was the case at the Cincinnati Children's Hospital, which is mentioned in the article. With regard to fish tanks, these provide a slice of nature and visual stimulation and can serve as a positive distraction (see Figure 4.04; also Figure 3.11). Presence of an aquarium has been shown to reduce anxiety in patients who were undergoing dental surgery.[23] These tanks must be maintained; they must be cleaned regularly (usually by a professional service); and care must be taken to make sure there are no dead fish![24]

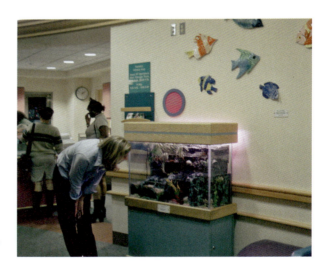

Figure 4.04: *Aquarium provides positive distraction, particularly for children.*
Location: Hasbro Children's Hospital, Providence, Rhode Island.

Windows, natural light, and views to nature as positive distractions

Everyday nature can positively impact health.[25] Essentially beginning with Ulrich's 1984 work, there is now a substantial literature on the health advantages of exposure to nature. Ulrich's initial study compared patients who had a view out their hospital room window to a brown brick wall or to everyday nature (a stand of deciduous trees). Those viewing nature had shorter post-operative stays and needed fewer doses of analgesics classified as either moderate or strong than did matched patients looking at the brick wall. As discussed in Chapter 1 in the context of outdoor garden spaces, the benefits of exposure to nature are numerous and have been linked to pain management; in addition, patients exposed to higher levels of light in their hospital rooms (as would have been the case for the patients in Ulrich's study looking at nature, not a wall), experienced less pain and reported a significantly greater decrease in stress at discharge.[26]

Views to nature can be provided in the waiting room (see Figure 1.12), in staff areas (see Figure 4.05), in the doctor's office, in consultation spaces, and even in exam rooms or treatment areas, such as those for infusion.

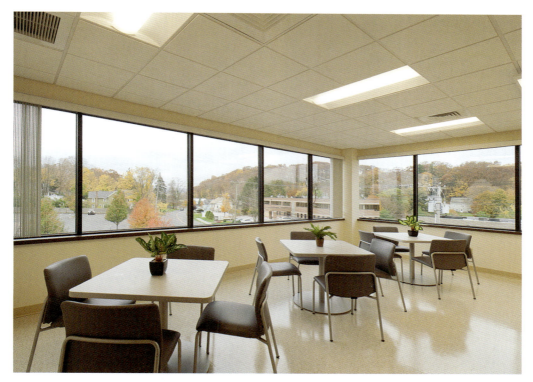

Figure 4.05: *Expansive windows with a view to nature for staff.*
Location: Western Connecticut Health Network, Pulmonary Relocation, Danbury, Connecticut.
Architect: The S/L/A/M Collaborative.
Photo credit: John Giammatteo

In the case of spaces where privacy is a primary consideration, curtains, blinds, or shades can be used but can be installed in such a way to leave light at the top, essentially to create a clerestory effect. When nature itself is not available, the simulation of nature through photographs, paintings, posters, and prints is recommended, with an emphasis on representational (not abstract) depictions of nature. A very effective example of this approach is shown in Figure 4.06, in which a firm used a screened print on a window shade to provide an alternative to what the patient would otherwise have seen – mechanical units in front of the treatment room windows. Dawn A. Gum, AIA, IIDA, a managing partner of the firm Interior Architecture & Design, PLLC, stated that "the concept for the project was based on 'borrowed views' as in a Japanese Garden" and "the silk screened tree on the window shade was the borrowed view in each treatment room."[27]

This approach to camouflaging an unattractive view has the potential to be used throughout healthcare facilities.

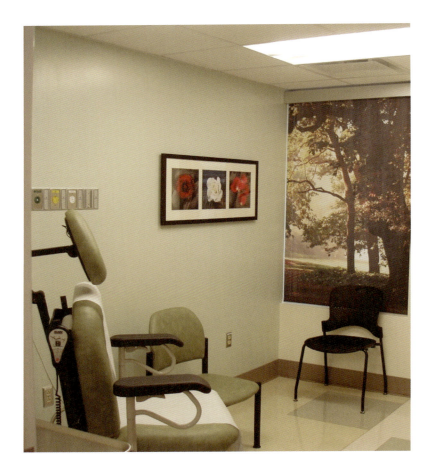

Figure 4.06: *Window screening both introduces nature and effectively hides mechanical equipment. Location: UNC Hospitals Wound Care Clinic, Chapel Hill, North Carolina. Architect: BBH Design and IDeA. Photo credit: Dawn A. Gum, AIA and IIDA*

Having windows in the waiting room to provide natural light is important; exposure to sunlight has been shown to improve mood.[28] Glare can be handled through drapes, shades, or blinds and also by using diffusers over fluorescent lamps or table lamps with incandescent bulbs.[29] Higher ceilings (10 ft vs. 8 ft) are typically associated with positive outcomes, such as an increase in creativity.[30] There is some suggestion that patients are more satisfied when the window occupies in the neighborhood of 20–30 percent of the window wall than when the window occupies a smaller percentage.[31]

In hospital interiors, Joey Fischer art images have been used to provide what is called visual therapy to create environments that contribute to the healing process.[32] Ceiling and wall murals of nature scenes are most often used in radiology and nuclear medicine areas, but the concepts can be transferred into the doctor's office. Imagine, for example, a mural of nature in the bathroom, on the wall of an examination room, or bringing the illusion of nature into a café through a virtual ceiling window, as in Figure 4.07.

The Ambient Environment 113

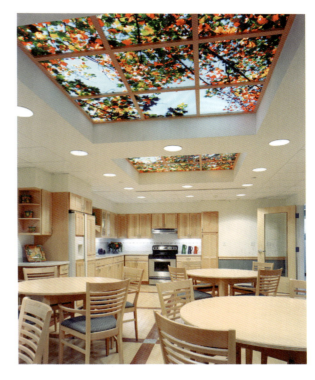

Figure 4.07: *Virtual ceiling window introduces nature into café.*
Location: Griffin Hospital, Inpatient Psychiatric Unit, Derby, Connecticut.
Architect: The S/L/A/M Collaborative.
Photo credit: Woodruff/Brown Architectural Photography

Restoration can also be provided through an activity like a labyrinth, the focus of the image on the right in Figure 4.08. The image on the left in that figure shows how it is possible to bring nature into the interior environment in a significant way. This image shows the interior courtyard that abuts the cafeteria of the Hospital da Luz (literally, of light) in Lisbon, Portugal.

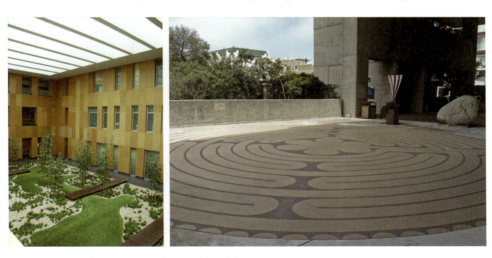

Figure 4.08: *Nature and restoration take a variety of forms.*
Location: Hospital da Luz, Lisbon, Portugal (left image); labyrinth at the California Pacific Medical Center, San Francisco, California (right image).

Access to nature for staff

Not having windows has an impact on office workers, and access to windows for administrative and clinical staff is important. In research on office workers in Norway, workers without windows were almost five times more likely to bring in plants and three times more likely to bring in pictures that depicted nature than were those with windows. This research is an advance over earlier studies on the topic as it controls for a variety of variables, including gender, age, view from the workspace itself, window view, and degree of personalization in the office.[33] Other research confirms this pattern of displaying more nature-oriented visual material in windowless offices than in windowed offices.[34]

When office workers from ten different complexes were surveyed regarding job stress and job satisfaction, those with a view to nature (a forested area) reported significantly higher job satisfaction and lower job stress, compared to those with a view to elements of the built environment (e.g., parking lots, other buildings). As the author argues, opportunities for passive exposure to nature, such as a view out a window, are important – especially given that active forms of stress release, such as exercise, are not always available.[35] Views of nature have been linked to stress reduction in a large number of studies.

Water as a positive distraction

The presence of water has a positive impact on humans, and the inclusion of water as a design feature in the outdoor landscape was mentioned in Chapter 1. A water feature can have a soothing effect and serve as a focal point in a reception area, as is evident in Figure 4.09.

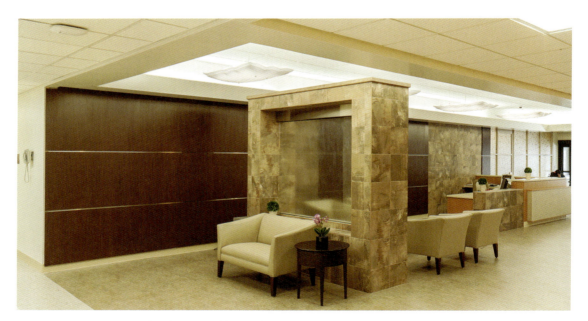

Figure 4.09: *Dramatic enclosed water wall in a lobby.*
Location: Clara Maass Medical Center, Continuing Care Building, Main Lobby, Belleville, New Jersey.
Architect: The S/L/A/M Collaborative.
Photo credit: John Giammatteo.

The Ambient Environment 115

Herzog makes the case that water compels us because it satisfies so many of the cognitive elements related to preference, including the ability to make sense of and be involved in the environment. Herzog argues that if your attention is fatigued, what will restore it is an expanse of smooth water.[36] Of importance in selecting art that could be shown in a waiting room, consultation room, or exam room is Herzog's finding that waterscape images that position the viewer at a distance from the element, taking a long view, are likely to be preferred.

This research provides a number of guidelines for using images in physicians' offices. First, the research underscores the positive response to nature and to water in particular. Second, it suggests that images need to be carefully selected; not every picture of nature is equally preferred. While it might be obvious that people are unlikely to prefer a picture of a swamp, it may not be as obvious that a waterfall might be more appreciated if the perspective presented in the picture is set at a distance. To some extent this recommendation fits with those of Ulrich and Gilpin[37] that turbulent water is to be avoided.

Water: A caution

Water elements such as small fountains are attractive in the waiting room and can provide both visual and auditory distraction; Yale-New Haven Hospital has used an indoor fountain in the atrium of its main hospital (seen in Figure 4.10) to great effect; the lobby of its Smilow Cancer Center also features a striking water wall. However, without proper installation or maintenance, such installations may pose a health hazard.[38] Fully enclosed waterscapes (refer to Figure 4.09) may be an alternative, but maintenance will still be an issue. If location permits, an alternative is a view to water in the landscape (see Figure 1.12).

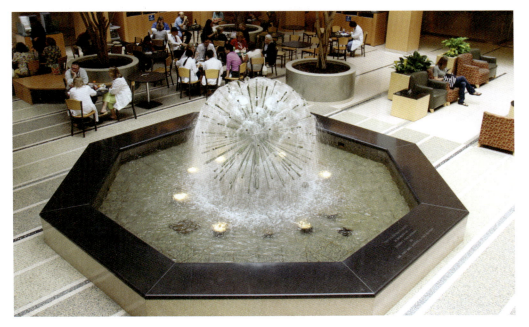

Figure 4.10: *Fountain provides a focal point in hospital atrium.*
Location: Atrium of the Yale-New Haven Hospital, New Haven, Connecticut.

Nature: The real deal

For many purposes in healthcare environments, simulated nature may be a reasonable substitute for the actual experience.[39] With regard to the viewing experience, a ten-minute nature film viewed on a large screen (72"), described as a more immersive environment, produced more pronounced recovery to stress on physiological responses than did watching the same film on a 31" screen. Thus, as the authors comment, when nature is not at hand, such immersive displays provide an alternative.[40] Often in healthcare settings rather modestly sized images are on display. This research suggests large images could be displayed to good effect. The painting in Figure 2.05, for example, is large enough to have an impact, as is the one in Figure 4.11.

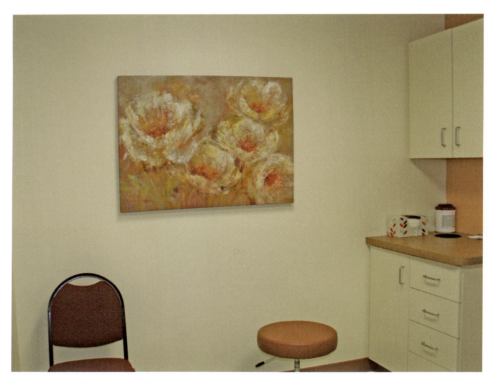

Figure 4.11: *Art provides positive distraction when it is large enough to have an impact. Location: Office of Neeraj Kohli, MD MBA, Wellesley, Massachusetts.*

The use of plants

Does it make a difference whether you use real plants or posters of plants? In research in a hospital waiting room, patients who were waiting in one of two hospital waiting rooms for a radiology service were exposed to: 1) live plants, 2) posters of nature, or 3) no nature. Patients rated perceived attractiveness of the waiting room and perceived stress. Patients reported significantly lower stress in both the poster and live nature conditions when compared to the no nature condition. Importantly, the attractiveness of the waiting room mediated the effect of the live plants and posters of plants. You cannot simply add plants or hang nature posters to reduce stress;

The Ambient Environment

the attractiveness of the waiting room matters as well.[41] If there are concerns about an increase in infections related to having live plants in the office, this research suggests that simulations of nature, for example through posters, may be adequate to reduce stress. In addition, entrances to offices can use plants to create a sense of welcome, as shown in Figure 4.12.

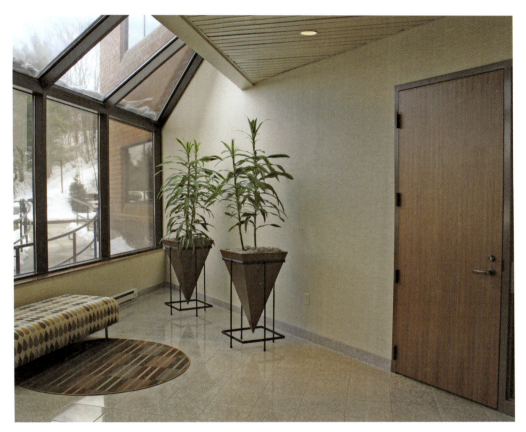

Figure 4.12: *Lobby landscaping and seating welcome patients. Location: Office of Neeraj Kohli, MD MBA, Wellesley, Massachusetts.*

Substitutes for nature: Art

Views of nature are restorative, but such views are not always available; a room may be windowless or provide a view of the built environment or mechanical equipment. Where views to nature are not available, photographs and paintings of nature can be substituted with some of the same results.[42] Images from Joey Fischer Art Research Institute Limited, a leader in the use of art in healthcare settings, were first used at Stanford.[43] Another resource is American Art Resources, a company whose mission is to "transform the healthcare environment through art."[44] Research consistently shows that representational art is preferred to abstract art; in particular, scenes of nature are preferred.[45] This preference holds across the developmental spectrum.[46] Abstract images, and images that are ambiguous or surreal, make people uncomfortable or anxious.[47]

The content of art: Recommendations

In Ulrich and Gilpin's summary of the literature, a primary consideration is that art be realistic (as opposed to abstract). The following categories are preferred: waterscapes (without turbulence); landscapes, with depth or an open foreground, lush vegetation, and cultural artifacts that are positively regarded (e.g., barns). In addition, flowers that look healthy (refer to Figure 4.11), figurative representations, in particular faces that depict positive emotion, scenes that show caring friendly relationships, and cultural diversity are recommended. Conversely, art images depicting ambiguity and chaotic forms with contrasting colors, and negative subject matter (e.g., threatening nature such as storms) are ill-advised.[48] Work by Hathorn and Nanda supports these recommendations.[49]

Too much of a good thing?

Has the value of positive distraction been oversold? Are too many visual distractions provided in healthcare settings? The Editor-in-Chief of *Healthcare Design* magazine offered an analysis in a blog titled "Killing the 'Visual Noise'"[50] – the argument made was to streamline the design in healthcare settings with the use of furniture in "simple solid colors" and uniform design. Maximizing whatever views to nature that already exist is preferable to visual overload.

The size of art: A comment

No guidelines have been offered, but it is worth noting that pictures in a waiting room have to be seen from across the room, which can be over 15 feet away. The details of small visual images are likely to be lost at that distance. Consideration should be given to larger murals of landscapes, whose content activates a schema (e.g., meadow; stream with covered bridge) (refer to Figure 2.05).

Visual microaggressions

Beyond the kind of art to display, its sociocultural aspects need to considered, otherwise a negative impact can occur. In a presentation a few years ago, I heard Derald Wing Sue, a psychologist well known for his writing on multiculturalism, talk about the concept of microaggression. Microaggressions are small slights or indignities that reflect negatively on a target, often a racial minority. Often these slights are unwitting, as in the example Dr. Sue offered, when he was told by a cab driver that he (Dr. Sue) spoke English very well. The cab driver's remark reflected his belief that no one who looked of Asian descent could speak English that well.

Microaggressions may come in visual form. Dr. Sue provided an example targeting Harvard College. Until the 2007 selection of Drew Faust, all Harvard presidents had been white men. How might a new faculty member of color feel, Dr. Sue asked, entering a room of presidential portraits in which there was no person who looked remotely like that faculty member? The faculty member was likely to feel unwelcome, in Dr. Sue's view. Thus, the physical environment itself can provide instances of microaggression, whether through the display of religious iconography that implicitly endorses one religion – signage only in English, or a myriad of other insensitivities. Every aspect of the visual environment should be evaluated in terms of its degree of welcomeness.

What you display affects patients

With regard to displays in the office, I am reminded of findings from two research projects; both indicate a lack of control about what is seen in medical offices can be upsetting. In a project on physicians' offices, participants rated the quality of care and comfort provided in 35 offices. The waiting room of one doctor had a display of swords on the wall, and one patient described these as "torture devices." We grouped this office with a number of others in the category "Strange and Uncomfortable" to describe the lack of comfort people felt in such environments.[51]

Similarly, the display of medical information, often on large posters, requires careful consideration. There is a difference between a medical poster that shows anatomy and one that depicts disease. Patients do not like the depiction of disease, as might be seen in photographs of skin lesions in a dermatologist's office. Such images could be illustrated just as easily in a medical pamphlet available to the patient. The difference between the poster and the pamphlet is the degree of personal control. Having a poster or photograph on the wall where it is hard to ignore is radically different from having a medical pamphlet that interested patients select for themselves. The act of selecting the pamphlet returns control to the patient.

In other research about experiences in doctors' offices, students were asked to provide positive and negative anecdotes about the office where they regularly received care.[52] One of the most common responses was that people did not like anatomical diagrams or displays of detailed medical information. Students preferred popular magazines and depictions of things to distract them, not to remind them of the impending exam, vaccination, or their symptoms. These quotations reflect this sentiment:

> I hate the examination room – white walls, medical themed wallpaper, posters of body parts, and pamphlets on diseases – yuck! It makes me feel so uncomfortable and I hate anxiously reading about AIDS or strep as I wait for the doctor to return.

> In-depth medical diagrams freak me out.

It is also noteworthy that, in this research, the participants had a far easier time generating examples of what they disliked than what they liked about the environment.

The displays of early practitioners: Implications for today

In early advice, practitioners were told that clues to character were reflected in their surroundings. Cathell warns the practitioner: "Let no sharks' heads, impaled butterflies, miniature ships, stuffed birds, or anything else be seen that will place you in any other light before patients than that of a physician."[53] Today, we are more aware of this association between what you display and who you are.[54] What, then, should today's physician display in the office?

Some advice from the past fits less well today, in particular the display of graphic references to disease. Such items as anatomical specimens and mementos from dissections were described by Cathell as appropriate and useful.[55] Their impact was to remind the patient of the physician's professional status, perhaps more necessary during a time when the status of the physician was less revered than today. There were regulars and irregulars (physicians who practiced unlicensed); knowledge and training in medicine was not yet standardized.

But consider this sage advice from author Wood in a chapter entitled "Some Essential Don'ts" in the classic *Dollars to Doctors* written in 1903. In this passage, the author highlights the negative effect displays can have on the patient:

> There is nothing handsomer than an exhibit of surgical instruments – that is to the general public – in a shop show window, or in a fair exhibit, but in a doctor's office they have a personal meaning, an indefinable feeling of dread fills a visitor at the paraphernalia of cutting and carving implements .... To make a pretentious display of them in a consulting room, is as bad as a grinning skull, or a rattling skeleton.[56]

Instead, what Wood suggests is a display of books which, he notes, inspire confidence and reflect positively on the physician's acquisition of knowledge. Wood has some wonderful examples of a physician who changed his office surroundings to reflect the season and make his patients feel more comfortable.[57]

Today, the profession is highly regulated, and rather than needing to be reminded of the physician's specialty by the display of artifacts, patients are often frightened by such displays – whether anatomical posters of the digestive system, photographs of skin lesions in a dermatologist's office, or even your own dental x-rays, now digitally displayed, facing you during dental cleanings.

Self-paced distraction: Reading material

Reading material, if it is current, appropriate for its audience, not dog-eared, and readily available, can be an important source of what is called self-paced distraction. In research on waiting rooms, when magazines and/or pamphlets were visible in the waiting room, that fact was commented upon positively.[58] In selecting reading materials, the clientele of the practice should be considered and an assortment of magazines should be offered. The general guidelines are: nothing offensive; a range of materials from classic news magazines (although these are now hard to find) to celebrity magazines like *People*; homemaker magazines like *Good Housekeeping*; sports-oriented magazines (e.g., like *Sports Illustrated*); and magazines focused on fashion, beauty, and hobbies. Subscription labels should be removed if staff members bring in magazines from home. Providing a place to store and display such material is important, as seen in Figure 4.13.

Figure 4.14 shows how literature can be neatly organized and housed in a patient and family resource area at Griffin Hospital in Derby, Connecticut. In their orientation to the facility, patients and family members would be shown the contents of the cabinets. Without such instruction, it is unlikely that people would feel they have permission to open the doors.

Music as positive distraction

A sizable literature shows the positive benefits of music, especially for pain management,[59] for patients undergoing and recovering from surgery;[60] but what evidence exists that playing music during a visit to an outpatient practitioner has benefits, for either patients or staff? A useful

The Ambient Environment 121

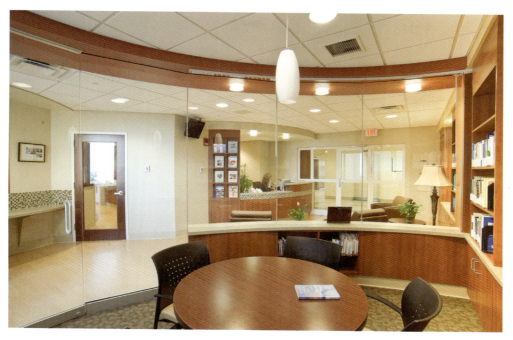

Figure 4.13: *Reading material on open shelving is accessible and neatly stored.*
Location: Bridgeport Hospital, Norma F. Pfriem Cancer Institute, Bridgeport, Connecticut.
Architect: The S/L/A/M Collaborative.
Photo credit: John Giammatteo

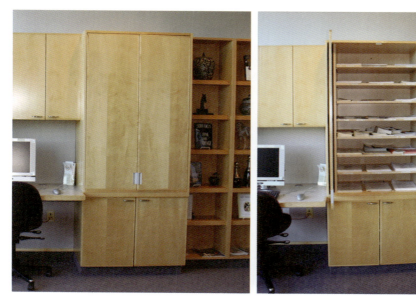

Figure 4.14: *Material can be stored behind closed doors, but patients need "permission" to look inside.*
Location: Patient and Family Resource Center, Griffin Hospital, Derby, Connecticut.

overview of the literature is provided by Dileo and Bradt,[61] who conducted a meta-analysis of medical music therapy. If we concentrate on outpatients and situations that could apply to office visits and waiting rooms, their meta-analysis shows that listening to music may enhance mood and/or decrease depression. Other research points to the use of music in reducing anxiety, reflected in 11 of 12 studies reviewed. There is some indication that it is preferable to let people use their own music, or at least be able to choose among selections.[62]

Preferred types of music

What kind of music should be played? Recommendations for music genre are light rock or jazz, which are unlikely to offend anyone.[63] Classical music has benefits, too.[64] Other research[65] has demonstrated that music can have a positive effect on arthritis pain when played for only 30 minutes. There is some evidence that when music accompanies nature (i.e., use of a nature videotape and music), the benefits in controlling pain are more pronounced.[66]

Sources of music: The CARE Channel (Continuous Ambient Relaxation Environment)

Susan Mazer is President and CEO of Healing HealthCare Systems® (HHS) in Reno, Nevada; her CARE Channel (Continuous Ambient Relaxation Environment) serves over "700 hospitals nationally," according to her vita. She and her partner Dallas Smith developed the CARE Channel as one way to reduce stress in healthcare settings. In a phone conversation with her in 2012, she noted it is a challenge to create music for a diverse population, with over 300 genres of music and up to four generations of family members potentially attending any given medical appointment.

In their book *Sound Choices: Using Music to Design the Environments in Which You Live, Work, and Heal*,[67] Mazer and Smith offer guidelines and pose questions for music in the healthcare environment: assess the sound environment, including sounds with sources outside the immediate room (such as others talking in a hallway); ask whether the music is appropriate (for patients they recommend music that will comfort and soothe and perhaps even inspire); ask whether the music fits the time of day, for example considering more up-tempo music at midday; ask how loud the room is, noting that "Every space has a volume."[68] A very good question they ask is whether the sound level fits the purpose of what goes on in the environment. "The role of the designer and architect is to prepare the space to minimize noise or unpleasant, erratic sounds and to support positive ones, such as music, necessary communications, patient privacy, and to facilitate staff effectiveness."[69]

Music: Mode of delivery and sources

Research has shown that music delivered by headphones and by loudspeakers both have the capacity to reduce the anxiety patients feel while waiting for surgery, in contrast to the results for a non-music control group.[70] In related research[71] patients listening to a light music genre via headphones had decreased stress, in terms of physiological measurement (decreased heart rate) as well as a subjective anxiety rating (on a visual analogue scale). If patients bring their own music and use earbuds, the concern about hygiene (due to the use of shared headphones) is reduced.

The Ambient Environment

A number of companies are emerging that market music to healthcare settings, including the French Music Care®[72] (www.music-care.com) as well as Healing Healthcare Systems®, which produces the CARE Channel that combines images of nature (landscapes, animals) with soothing music that can be used in waiting areas.[73] Healthcare practitioners could use radio stations, but then commercials would be heard unless they use satellite stations, like Sirius, which play few or no ads. If you broadcast CDs in a public environment, you must pay copyright fees to BMI or ASCAP.

Exercising control: Having patients bring their own music

Brief exposure to music appears to have a self-reported relaxation effect. Moreover, if people are encouraged to bring their own music selections (e.g., on an iPod), this approach also enhances their sense of control. Other research has also pointed to the control provided by listening to one's own music in situations where pain tolerance is an issue.[74] Practitioners might encourage patients to bring their own music. At the same time, other research shows it is possible to provide music that is pleasing to a large percentage (82 percent) of patients.[75]

In summary, the practical implication of the research on music in healthcare environments seems to be that "Music intervention is safe, inexpensive and easily used to improve the healing environment."[76]

Complimentary food and beverages

Food and odor are combined pleasantly in Planetree facilities, where visitors as well as patients may be served beverages and offered fresh baked goods, the smell of which often permeates the facility. In addition to pleasant odors, such smells can often overpower the institutional smells often associated with healthcare settings. In addition, lobby and reception spaces can offer healthy snacks.[77]

One of the first aspects of the waiting rooms mentioned to me by a good friend who needed to consult a specialist was the complimentary beverage area (see Figure 4.15). In this example, the area is encountered first as you enter the office suite. A single-serve coffee maker is used, which may: 1) produce better coffee over the course of the day, and 2) facilitate neatness. My friend said the area was immaculate and welcoming. Another effective example is shown in Figure 4.16, which again employs a single-serve coffee brewer. The area need not be large to be effective; in some respects, a smaller area might constrain litter.

In her commentary describing positive distractions during a wait in a medical facility, Caroline Leemis[78] mentions the idea of a small café area; this in essence is what welcomed my friend arriving for her appointment. Dietrick et al.[79] found that access to food was important to family members in an intensive care unit waiting room and influenced their judgments of the services provided. Patients and family members in the waiting room of a practitioner's office are generally not experiencing the same level of stress as if they were visiting an inpatient; it is nevertheless a courtesy and a kindness to consider beverages and packaged (not open) snacks. Even a vending machine offering nutritious snacks and water, perhaps in the entry area, could be considered. Access to water is recommended by patients who were asked to suggest improvements to waiting rooms.[80]

The Ambient Environment

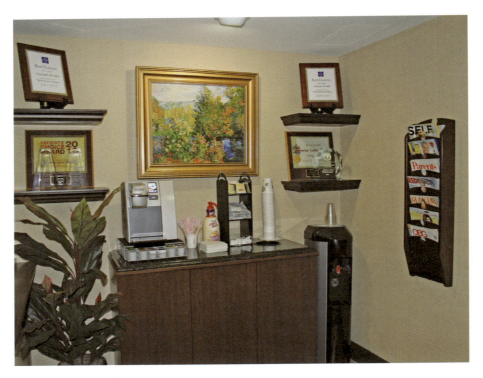

Figure 4.15: *Welcoming complimentary beverage center.*
Location: Office of Neeraj Kohli, MD MBA, Wellesley, Massachusetts.

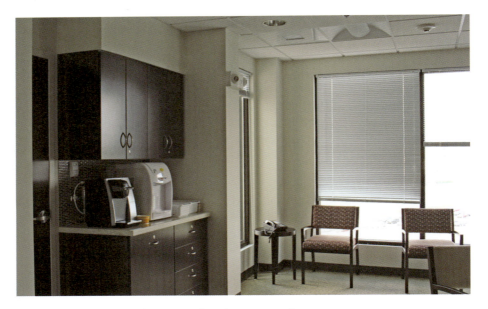

Figure 4.16: *Single-brew coffee machine streamlines beverage service.*
Location: Women & Infants Center for Reproduction and Infertility, Providence, Rhode Island.

Other senses

Cleanliness and odor

Cleanliness matters, and patients notice. In research in the United Kingdom, comparing ratings patients left on a National Health Service website called NHS Choices, better ratings of hospital cleanliness (on a scale from 1 = dirty to 5 = exceptionally clean) were in fact associated with lower rates of infection from methicillin-resistant *Staphylococcus aureus* (MRSA);[81] the case is made that cleanliness does matter, as does the patient's evaluation of the environment.[82]

In a healthcare setting, the degree of cleanliness is indicated by such physical traces as the previous patient's debris (e.g., a soiled gown on an examination table), poor maintenance (e.g., un-emptied trash), marks, dings, and the smell of sickness. When patients in an emergency department were asked about factors that influenced satisfaction, the air smell was an important component.[83] In his book on research tools in design, John Zeisel devotes one chapter to physical traces;[84] he discusses how what we leave behind, the detritus, typically indicates some failure of design. When debris is left on an exam table or instruments not shelved, it may be that the design does not support the function of the space. If there are stains, dirty baseboards, and smells, we may be concerned about cleanliness and upkeep.[85] Pathogens that are problematic usually come from the people in the building. For that reason, such preventative measures as effective air filters, hand sanitizers, and furnishings that can be cleaned are important.

Hand-washing is the most effective step to reduce the transmission of disease.[86] An intervention study in England reminded people to wash their hands with a "clean your hands" campaign with posters and marketing materials, including those for patients. In addition, NPAHs (near-patient alcohol hand rubs) were added. The multi-method approach to improve hand-washing significantly increased compliance.[87] Alcohol hand rub use increased by 184 percent, with increased compliance reported by 74 percent of staff. Information related to training and management, including how to obtain posters that could be posted for office staff, is readily available from the Center for Disease Control.[88]

Air quality and odor

Among the issues to consider are ventilation, relative humidity, and smell.[89] Patients surveyed in 17 different waiting areas were asked to rate the quality of the physical environment.[90] Air freshness appeared on a number of dimensions, as did temperature, a related variable. Patients were more satisfied with cleanliness in the morning than in the afternoon, pointing to the need for frequent cleaning of the restrooms (e.g., emptying of trash). Indoor air quality can be addressed through the frequency of air changes per hour (ACH), and physicians should consult with contractors/maintenance people to determine the adequacy of the ACH in the waiting area. Guidelines for ventilation standards are available from a number of sources, including the American Institute of Architects and the American Society of Heating, Refrigerating, and Air-conditioning Engineers (ASHRAE), although there is no firm determination about the minimum requirements to prevent disease.

Aromatherapy

Aromatherapy is the therapeutic use of essential oils extracted from plants. This approach has a relatively long history in Europe.[91] Relaxation may be associated with smelling particular essential oils such as lavender, often in the form of oils used in massage, but the use of such fragrances in any substantial way may not be welcomed by those with various kinds of allergies and sensitivities. The real focus should be on the cleanliness of the environment and, in keeping with the greening of the environment, the use of cleaning materials that are environmentally friendly.

Noxious fumes are obviously to be avoided in healthcare settings (and elsewhere), but on the other hand, unfortunately, we know little about the effects of adding pleasant smells to the environment. Use of orange essential oil in the waiting room of a dental practice affected women but not men. The women were positively affected in terms of increased calmness and elevated mood; further, pre-treatment state anxiety was lowered.[92]

What happens when you use an odorant that is diffused? Finding no studies of aromatherapy on large groups, Holm and Fitzmaurice[93] studied the effects of music and aromatherapy (either alone or in combination) in a pediatric referral center. A system of loudspeakers in the waiting room broadcast classical music; the aromatherapy was from an essential oil derived from an orange blossom (Neroli). Two diffusers, at opposite ends of the waiting room, dispensed the scent every 30–60 minutes during the study. The music decreased self-reported anxiety; the aromatherapy did not. The authors comment that the diffusers may have been too weak against the backdrop of the hospital airflow system to circulate air continuously.

Temperature and thermal comfort

People are unhappy when the temperature is too hot or too cold; in research on emergency departments, temperature extremes bothered patients more than crowding, messiness, poor air quality, or poor wayfinding information (signage). Patient satisfaction and willingness to recommend to others are related to room temperature, among other variables.[94] As noted in Chapter 3, exam room temperatures where people are partially clothed should be higher than in consultation spaces.

Cleanliness and carpeting

The use of carpeting in inpatient settings is controversial,[95] but research has demonstrated that vancomycin-resistant enterococci (VRE), antimicrobial-resistant bacteria, are less likely to survive on carpeting than on materials often used in healthcare settings such as vinyl composition flooring, rubber tile, or linoleum.[96] The advantages of carpeting in noise reduction and the communication of home-like qualities make it the recommended choice in doctors' offices. With the exception of the bathroom or where spills are likely to be a major concern, carpeting can be used throughout the suite of rooms.[97] Darker colors and/or those with a pattern are more likely to resist showing dirt and stains; the use of patterns provides an opportunity to add visual interest, as seen in Figure 4.17.

Carpeting that is antimicrobial and antistatic with a backing that is impermeable is recommended.[98] Carpeting should be inspected routinely to make sure there are no frayed areas or looseness that might lead to tripping and falling.

The Ambient Environment 127

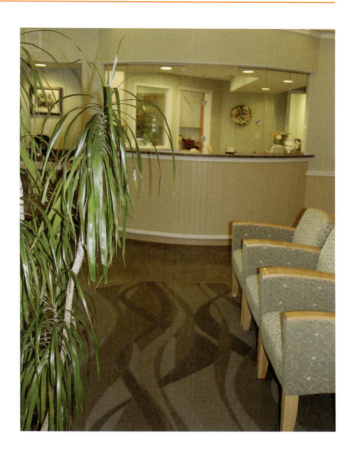

Figure 4.17: *A dark patterned carpet resists stains and provides visual interest. Location: Coastal Connecticut Dentistry, Waterford, Connecticut.*

Green cleaning and design

The environment must be clean because cleanliness matters in patient satisfaction as well as health outcomes; the question is how to clean the environment in the least harmful way. Given the desire to protect the environment, a topic garnering recent attention is green cleaning, which focuses on how to improve health in the environment – for example, by reducing HAIs without harming the environment. A white paper from the Healthier Hospitals Initiative's Pebble Project from the Center for Health Design addresses the issue of green cleaning.[99] This topic has ramifications in the doctor's office, where patients and staff may be exposed to chemicals in cleaning products. At the scale of the doctor's office, harmful chemicals can be ingredients of window cleaners, general-purpose cleaners, as well as bathroom cleaners. Dermatitis from such products can affect both patients and staff, and those who have asthma and who are pregnant can be impacted as well.

What are the ramifications from a design perspective? The white paper provided a conceptual framework of green cleaning issues in healthcare. Building components that apply to the practitioner's office are the ventilation system, the surface finish of materials, technology (e.g., automated faucets), and furnishings. Accommodation for waste management and recycling is also relevant. Layout and selection of materials, especially flooring, are important. One layout issue mentioned is the location of the housekeeping closet, which could affect efficiency and cleaning time.

With regard to selecting flooring material, recommendations include rubber flooring, large ceramic tiles with little grout, attractive wood-looking linoleum sheet vinyl instead of vinyl composition tile (VCT) flooring that requires stripping and waxing on a regular basis, and vinyl-free resilient flooring. Green Seal cleaners are mentioned as simultaneously providing adequate cleaning while protecting the environment. Their website lists green cleaning products for industrial and institutional use.[100] Herman Miller, Inc. also has useful research summaries on environmental design, including green issues in healthcare environments. Their article "Healthier Planet, Healthier People: Hospitals Go Green to 'First Do No Harm'"[101] provides recommendations to reduce mercury and the use of PVCs in the environment. Another excellent source of information is the organization Health Care Without Harm whose goal is to create ecologically sustainable healthcare settings that cause no harm to either people or the environment (see www.noharm.org). Their website lists numerous fact sheets on green purchasing tools and resources, organized by global geographical sector. Another resource is Green Guidelines for Healthcare, which emphasizes "sustainable building design, construction, and operations for the healthcare industry."[102]

Safety in the medical suite: By regulation and by association

A host of regulations exist to guide the creation of safe environments, including those from ADA legislation and OSHA. These guidelines create safety by regulation. Safety by association capitalizes on people's experiences with the environment or their schemas of how the environment is typically structured for safety. There are times when design may conform to regulation but run counter to experience or limit options (e.g., when the parking lot meets regulations but provides limited turning options for elderly drivers). The safest environments occur when safety by association coincides with safety by regulation. Advocates for universal design often make the case that universal design standards that address a range of challenges (e.g., of mobility) ultimately improve the environment for everyone. Similarly, thinking beyond regulations to people's expectations regarding environmental design (e.g., that a coat rack would be weighted on the bottom and not likely to tip over) can lead to improved safety standards for everyone. That viewpoint is endorsed here.

Safety by design

Exhaustive coverage of safety related to design is beyond the scope of this book, but a selection of aspects will be mentioned. One of these is falls – a major source of injury in the United States, particularly among those aged 65 and older.[103][104][105][106] A good overview of the relationship between environmental design and falls by patients is provided by Gulwadi and Calkins.[107]

Many of the safety practices recommended for inpatient units can be applied to the practitioner's office. These include considering the properties of flooring, including "floor type (carpet vs. resilient), its finish (polished, high-gloss) and other properties (how absorbent or how slippery when wet)."[108] Commercial-grade, low-pile, and tightly woven carpeting without highly contrasting patterns is recommended in the context of assisted living facilities and nursing homes. These recommendations apply more broadly, in my view. Particular attention should be given to the transitions of flooring type where cane tips or crutches could catch. Other recommendations that could apply to the practitioner's office include evenness of lighting levels to eliminate shadows.

Falls can occur in a practitioner's office as well as on an inpatient unit, but so can electrocution by exposed bare wires on an aquarium in an internist's office! A useful checklist is provided in an article about spotting safety hazards in the office.[109] The article also provides sources for safety regulations and a checklist to use for evaluating safety conditions. A 2009 white paper devoted to enhancing safety and quality, issued by the Institute for Healthcare Improvement in Cambridge, Massachusetts, is useful.[110] Huisman, Morales, van Hoof, and Kort[111] provide a very good overview of health risks related to the physical environment of healthcare settings and offer recommendations in each of their sections. Patient safety also relates to patient identity in the form of protecting HIPAA information. OfficeWorks™, a medical staffing organization, provides useful recommendations to safeguard patient personal health information (e.g., relating to HIPAA Compliance, Work Place Safety, and Universal Precautions).[112] Safety by Design, which includes patient and environmental safety in addition to worker and workplace safety, has been incorporated by Kaiser Permanente, the largest not-for-profit health plan.[113]

A useful article entitled "Spot the Safety Hazards in This Office – and Yours"[114] reminds us that making the office safe is a daily challenge. Analysis of the recommendations in the article indicates that having sufficient storage emerges as a theme. Sufficient storage can prevent putting boxes in places that can impede egress in a fire or on high shelves, which can lead to possible head injuries. Sufficient storage also relates to the separation of waste and safe storage of cleaning supplies.

Safety issues, which the article lists, are present in the exterior environment as well. These safety issues include keeping walkways and driveways free of debris; trimming trees to clear them from contact with overhead wires; making sure exterior lights and lighted signs operate. The article points readers to other sources of information about safety, including materials from the Emergency Care Research Institute,[115] which offers Physician Office Fundamentals in Risk Management and Patient Safety. Other useful resources are available from the Agency for Research Healthcare and Quality, particularly their materials on Quality and Patient Safety.

Functionality and safety: Related concerns

Accidents happen when design fails to accommodate typical behavior. One approach to functionality is to think about what we have at home that needs to be accommodated in the doctor's office. We need a place to hang coats, which is often overlooked. In one medical practice the receptionist often tells patients to put their coats on the bamboo stalks, a decorative feature in the front hall, because there is no coat closet. We also need a place for wet umbrellas; we need a drink of water; we need trash receptacles; we need enough space for walkers, wheelchairs, and strollers; we need clean air; and we need a place for children.

Many useful ideas to address these and other functionalities and improve safety and patients' experience in the doctor's office are provided by Fuelfor, a design company in Barcelona.[116] Their solutions range from including air-cleaning plants to queue displays at the end of each seating area and on handheld devices. Other ideas include storage areas for walkers, wheelchairs, strollers; providing a play area for children separated from the adult area with a low panel; cushions that are comfortable yet hygienic; vending machines with healthy choices and nutritional information offered in a way to encourage interaction, rather than passive consumption. With regard to providing complimentary beverages, even staid institutions like libraries are changing (e.g., "Would you like a latte with that library card?")[117] Providing complimentary beverages is another way to communicate the level of care that is provided, as shown in Figures 4.15 and 4.16. Other functionalities that should be provided in the waiting room include a clock, calendar, computers with a screen saver visible (to indicate the computer is turned on), and seating at a height appropriate to use this technology.

Closing Thoughts

One of the lessons in this book is that schemas matter. The schema of materials used in healthcare is changing, precipitated by the Planetree movement and the rise of consumerism in all aspects of health. Another theme is the role of competency, choice, and the opportunity for control in the healthcare setting. These aspects are important because they can help reduce stress. Healthcare settings provoke tremendous anxiety, even for routine care. Stress can be reduced through an effective wayfinding program; finding your way can provide a sense of competence. Stress can also be reduced by giving patients some control, whether in terms of keeping themselves clothed during much of the visit, or providing technology for them to use in the waiting area. Stress can also be reduced through positive distractions. As this chapter indicates, investing care in an environment through a host of positive distractions yields significant benefits to the patient and the practice.

In a recent *New York Times* column entitled "House of Death," the author, an internist, writes about avoiding the actual physical environment of an inpatient hospice unit, although she had never been inside one.[118] Her expectations or schema about the building, the "shared physical space and sheer number of people dying in it at once," created a dread that almost prevented her from visiting her dying patient. Much to her surprise, inside it was "quiet, and cozy, and homey" – not at all what she expected; rather, her impression was of a "radiant place" that provided a supportive environment for the end of life. The physical environment does matter, as the research featured in this book has shown. We have the evidence we need to transform healthcare spaces.

Further Reading

American Art Resources: Transforming the Healthcare Experience Through Art. Homepage: http://www.americanartresources.com/index.htm
Center for Disease Control and Prevention. "Hand Hygiene in Healthcare Settings." Center for Disease Control and Prevention. http://www.cdc.gov/handhygiene/
CrockettSTUDIO, "TV's in the Waiting Room? A Design Dilemma," CrockettSTUDIO. http://crockettstudio.wordpress.com/2011/03/24/tvs-in-the-waiting-room-a-design-dilemma/
Gaerig, Chris. "Televisions in Waiting Rooms," *Healthcare Design*, June 15, 2010. http://www.healthcaredesignmagazine.com/blogs/cgaerig/televisions-waiting-rooms
Green Seal. Homepage: http://www.greenseal.org/AboutGreenSeal.aspx
Hathorn, Kathy, and Upali Nanda. "A Guide to Evidence-Based Art." The Center for Health Design, March, 2008. http://www.healthdesign.org/sites/default/files/Hathorn_Nanda_Mar08.pdf
HermanMiller Healthcare. "Healthier Planet, Healthier People: Hospitals Go Green to 'First Do No Harm.'" http://www.hermanmiller.com/content/dam/hermanmiller/documents/research_summaries/wp_GreenHospitals.pdf
Huisman, E. R. C. M., Ester J. Morales, Joost Van Hoof, and Helianthe S. M. Kort. "Healing Environment: A Review of the Impact of the Physical Environment." *Building and Environment* 58, (2012): 70–80.

Leemis, Caroline. "ASID: Providing Positive Distractions During the Patient Wait Experience." *Healthcare Design*, June 13, 2010. http://www.healthcaredesignmagazine.com/blogs/acleemis/asid-providing-positive-distractions-during-patient-wait-experience

Lowes, Robert. "Spot the Safety Hazards in This Office – and Yours." *Medical Economics*, May 7, 2001. http://medicaleconomics.modernmedicine.com/medical-economics/news/spot-safety-hazards-office-and-yours

Lowes, Robert. "Starting a Practice 5–6 Months Out: Office Design and Supplies." *Medical Economics*, June 18, 2004. http://medicaleconomics.modernmedicine.com/medical-economics/news/clinical/practice-management/starting-practice5-6-months-out-office-design-an

Mazer, Susan E. "Music and Nature at the Bedside: Part One of a Two-Part Series." *Research Design Connections*, Issue 4, (2009). http://healinghealth.com/images/uploads/files/Music_and_Nature_at_the_Bedside-_Part_One_of_a_Two-part_Series__Research_Design_Connections.pdf

Mazer, Susan E. "Music and Nature at the Bedside: Part II of a Two-Part Series. *Research Design Connections*, Issue 1, (2010). http://healinghealth.com/images/uploads/files/MusicNature_at_the_Bedside-Part_2.pdf

Mazer, Susan, and Dallas Smith, *Sound Choices: Using Music to Design the Environments in Which You Live, Work, and Heal*. Carlsbad, CA: Hay House, Inc., 1999.

OfficeWorks™. "HIPAA Compliance, Work Place Safety, and Universal Precautions." OffceWorks™: A Medical Staffing Organization. Accessed August 1, 2013. http://www.officeworksrx.com/documents/HIPAAUniversalPrecautionsSafety.pdf

Quan, Xiaobo, Anjali Joseph, and Matthew Jelen. "Green Cleaning in Healthcare: Current Practices and Questions for Future Research." The Center for Health Design, September, 2011. http://www.healthdesign.org/chd/research/green-cleaning-healthcare-current-practices-and-questions-future-research

Sadler, Blair L., Anjali Joseph, Amy Keller, and Bill Rostenberg. "Using Evidence-Based Environmental Design to Enhance Safety and Quality." IHI Innovation Series White Paper. Cambridge, Massachusetts: Institute for Healthcare Improvement. Last modified April 24, 2011. http://www.ihi.org/knowledge/Pages/IHIWhitePapers/UsingEvidenceBasedEnvironmentalDesignWhitePaper.aspx

Stuckey, Heather L., and Jeremy Nobel. "The Connection between Art, Healing, and Public Health: A Review of Current Literature." *American Journal of Public Health* 100(2), (2010): 254–263.

The CARE Channel. Resources: http://healinghealth.com/resources-main/

Ulrich, Roger S. "View Through a Window May Influence Recovery from Surgery." *Science* 224, (1984): 420–421. doi:10.1126/science.6143402

Ulrich, Roger, and Laura Gilpin. "Healing Arts: Nutrition for the Soul." In *Putting Patients First: Designing and Practicing Patient-Centered Care*, edited by Susan B. Frampton, Laura Gilpin, and Patrick A. Charmel, 117–146. San Francisco, CA: Jossey-Bass, 2003.

Ulrich, Roger S., Craig Zimring, Xuemei Zhu, Jennifer DuBose, Hyun-Bo Seo, Young-Seon Choi, Xiaobo Quan, and Anjali Joseph. "A Review of the Research Literature on Evidence-Based Healthcare Design." *Health Environments Research & Design Journal* 1, (Spring 2008): 61–125.

Zeisel, John. *Inquiry by Design: Tools for Environment-Behavior Research*. Monterey, CA: Brooks/Cole Publishing, 1981.

Notes

Introduction

1. Cathell, Daniel Webster. *The Physician Himself and What He Should Add to His Scientific Acquirements.* New York: Arno Press & *The New York Times*, 1882/1972, 14.
2. Hess, Alice Jo. *History of Medicine in Harrison County West Virginia.* Parson, WV: McClain Printing Company, 1978, 22.
3. Cathell, *The Physician Himself*, 10.
4. Mathews, Joseph McDowell. *How to Succeed in the Practice of Medicine*. Philadelphia: W. B. Saunders & Company, 1905, 46.
5. Cathell, *The Physician Himself*, 21–22.
6. Gosling, Sam. *Snoop: What Your Stuff Says About You.* New York: Basic Books, 2009.
7. Carr, Robert F. "Health Care Facilities." National Institute of Building Sciences. Last modified December 30, 2010. http://www.wbdg.org/design/health_care.php
8. Chebat, Jean-Charles, M. Joseph Sirgy, and Valerie St. James. "Upscale Image Transfer from Malls to Stores: A Self-Image Congruence Explanation." *Journal of Business Research* 59(12), (2006): 1288–1296. doi:10.1016/j.jbusres.2006.09.007
9. Planetree. "Planetree Pioneers: Angelica Thieriot." Planetree. Accessed August 1, 2013. http://planetree.org/?page_id=68
10. Devlin, Ann Sloan. "Staff, Patients, and Visitors: Responses to Hospital Unit Enhancements." In *26th Environmental Design Research Association Conference Proceedings,* edited by Jack L. Nasar, Peg Grannis, and Kazunari Hanyu, 113–117. Oklahoma City, OK: Environmental Design Research Association, 1995; Martin, Diane P., Julie R. Hunt, Mary Hughes-Stone, and Douglas A. Conrad. "The Planetree Model Hospital Project: An Example of the Patient as Partner." *Hospital & Health Services Administration* 35, (1990): 591–601.
11. Stone, Susan. "A Retrospective Evaluation of the Impact of the Planetree Patient-centered Model of Care on Inpatient Quality Outcomes." *Health Environments Research and Design Journal* 1(4), (Summer 2008): 55–69.
12. Charmel, Patrick A. "Building the Business Case for Patient-centered Care." In *Putting Patients First: Designing and Practicing Patient-Centered Care*, edited by Susan. B. Frampton, Laura Gilpin, and Patrick. A. Charmel, 193–204. San Francisco: Jossey-Bass, 2003.
13. Michael Romano. "Personal Space." *Modern Healthcare* 35(31), (August 1, 2005): 20.
14. Institute for Healthcare Improvement. "Idealized Design of Clinical Office Practices." Institute for Healthcare Improvement, July, 2000. http://clinicalmicrosystem.org/materials/worksheets/IDCOP_Guide.pdf
15. Henriksen, Kerm, Sandi Isaacson, Blair L. Sadler, and Craig Zimring. "The Role of the Physical Environment in Crossing the Quality Chasm." *The Joint Commission Journal on Quality and Patient Safety* 33(11) supplement, (2007): 68–80.
16. Practice Greenhealth. "History." Practice Greenhealth. Accessed August 1, 2013. http://practicegreenhealth.org/about/history
17. Healthcare Construction and Operations. "Ft. Belvoir Replacement Hospital Nears Completion." Healthcare Construction and Operations, June 11, 2010. http://www.hconews.com/articles/2010/06/11/ft-belvoir-replacement-hospital-nears-completion

18 Reuters. "More Than Half of Americans Use Internet for Health." Reuters, February 3, 2010. http://www.reuters.com/article/2010/02/03/us-internet-health-idUSTRE6120HM20100203
19 Marquardt, Gesine, and Tom Motzek. "How to Rate the Quality of a Research Paper: Introducing a Helpful Algorithm for Architects and Designers." *Health Environments Research & Design* (Winter 2013): 119–127.
20 Kaplan, Stephen, and Rachel Kaplan. *Humanscape: Environments for People.* North Scituate, MA: Duxbury Press, 1978; Kaplan, Stephen, and Rachel Kaplan. *Cognition and Environment: Functioning in an Uncertain World.* New York: Praeger, 1982.
21 White, Robert. "Motivation Reconsidered: The Concept of Competence." *Psychological Review* 66(5), (1959): 297–333.
22 Seligman, Martin E. P. *Helplessness: On Depression, Development, and Death.* San Francisco: W. H. Freeman, 1975; Seligman, Martin E. P., and Steven F. Maier. "Failure to Escape Traumatic Shock." *Journal of Experimental Psychology* 74(1), (1967): 1–9. doi:10.1037/h0024514
23 Altman, Irwin. *The Environment and Social Behavior: Privacy, Personal Space, Territoriality, Crowding.* Monterey, CA: Brooks/Cole Publishing Company, 1975.
24 Sommer, Robert. *Personal Space.* Englewood Cliffs, NJ: Prentice Hall, 1969.

Chapter 1

1 Church, Thomas D., Grace Hall, and Michael Laurie, *Gardens are for People*, 2nd ed. New York: McGraw-Hill Book Company, 1983, 65.
2 Miller, George. A. "The Magical Number Seven, Plus or Minus Two: Some Limits on Our Capacity for Processing Information." *Psychological Review* 63(2), (1956): 81–97. doi:10.1037/h0043158
3 Cowan, Nelson. "The Magical Number 4 in Short-Term Memory: A Reconsideration of Mental Storage Capacity." *The Behavioral and Brain Sciences* 24(1), (2001): 87–185. doi:10.1017/S0140525X01003922
4 Ophir, Eyal, Clifford Nass, and Anthony D. Wagner. "Cognitive Control in Media Multitasks." *PNAS Proceedings of the National Academy of Sciences of the United States of America* 106, (2009): 15583–15587. doi:10.1073/pnas.0903620106
5 Borst, Grégoire, William L. Thompson, and Stephen M. Kosslyn. "Understanding the Dorsal and Ventral Systems of the Human Cerebral Cortex." *American Psychologist* 66(7), (2011): 624–632. doi:10.1037/a0024038
6 Davis, Dorothy. *History of Harrison County, West Virginia*, edited by Elizabeth Sloan. Clarksburg, WV: American Association of University Women, 1970. This book contains references to a paper read by my paternal grandfather at a meeting of the 50-year club, March 19, 1952. My aunt edited the book, which may explain why my grandfather appears so prominently in the chapter on Medicine. Herbert Elias Sloan, MD "Clarksburg Doctors Fifty Years Ago." *Fifty Year Club Papers.* Clarksburg, WV: Harrison County Historical Society, 1953.
7 Cathell, *The Physician Himself*, 27, (see Introduction, n. 1).
8 Starr, Paul. *The Social Transformation of American Medicine.* New York: Basic Books, Inc. Publishers, 1982, 22.
9 Arneill, Allison, and Ann Sloan Devlin. "Perceived Quality of Care: The Influence of the Waiting Room Environment." *Journal of Environmental Psychology* 22(4), (2002): 345–360. doi:10.1006/jevp.2002.0274
10 Davis, *History of Harrison County*, 499.
11 Helpful sources on this topic: American Hospital Association. *Signs and Graphics for Health Care Facilities.* Chicago: American Hospital Publishing, Inc., 1979; Berger, Craig. *Wayfinding: Designing and Implementing Graphic Navigation Systems.* Hove, UK: RotoVision SA, 2005.
12 Rosner, David. *A Once Charitable Enterprise: Hospitals and Health Care in Brooklyn and New York, 1885–1915.* New York, Cambridge University Press, 1982, 30.

Notes

13 Cathell, *The Physician Himself*, 10.
14 Marks, Barbara. "The Language of Signs." In *Sign Systems for Libraries*, edited by Dorothy Pollet and Peter C. Haskell, 91. New York: R. R. Bowker Co., 1979.
15 American Hospital Association, *Signs and Graphics*, 2.
16 Marks, *Language*, 91.
17 Cooper, Randy. *Wayfinding for Health Care: Best Practices for Today's Facilities*. Chicago: HealthForum, Inc., 2010, 2–12.
18 Sloane, David Charles, and Beverlie Conant Sloane, *Medicine Moves to the Mall*. Baltimore: The Johns Hopkins University Press, 2003, 167.
19 Lynch, Kevin. *The Image of the City*. Cambridge, MA: The MIT Press, 1960.
20 See for example, Trulove, James Grayson, Connie Sprague, and Steel Colony. *This Way: Signage Design for Public Spaces*. Gloucester, MA: Rockport Publishers, 2000.
21 Cooper, *Wayfinding*, 12.
22 Cooper, *Wayfinding*, 12.
23 Cohen, Aaron, and Elaine Cohen. "Architectural Techniques for Wayfinding." In *Sign Systems for Libraries*, edited by Dorothy Pollet and Peter C. Haskell, 187–193. New York: R. R. Bowker Co., 1979.
24 Downs, Roger M. "Mazes, Minds, and Maps." In *Sign Systems for Libraries*, edited by Dorothy Pollet and Peter C. Haskell, 17–32. New York: R. R. Bowker Co., 1979.
25 Weisman, Gerald. "Improving Wayfinding and Architectural Legibility in Housing for the Elderly." In *Housing the Aged: Design Directives and Policy Considerations*, edited by Victor Regnier and Jon Pynoos, 441–464. New York: Elsevier, 1987; see also Carpman, Janet Reizenstein, Myron R. Grant, and Deborah A. Simmons. *Design that Cares: Planning Health Facilities for Patients and Visitors*. Chicago: American Hospital Publishing, Inc., 1986.
26 See Calori, 78–81, for a detailed discussion of these issues. Calori, Chris. *Signage and Wayfinding Design: A Complete Guide to Creating Environmental Graphic Design Systems*. Hoboken, NJ: John Wiley & Sons, Inc., 2007.
27 For a full discussion of these issues, see: Smitshuijzen, Edo. *Signage Design Manual*. Baden, Switzerland: Lars Müller Publishers, 2007.
28 Mathews, *How to Succeed*, 40, (see Introduction, n. 4).
29 Cathell, *The Physician Himself*, 12.
30 Uebele, Andreas. *Signage Systems & Information Graphics: A Professional Sourcebook*. New York: Thames & Hudson, 2007.
31 Wilt, Lawrence J. M., and Jane Maienschein. "Symbol Signs for Libraries." In *Sign Systems for Libraries*, edited by Dorothy Pollett and Peter C. Haskell, 108. New York: R. R. Bowker Co., 1979.
32 Selfridge, Katherine M. "Planning Library Signage Systems." In *Sign Systems for Libraries*, edited by Dorothy Pollet and Peter C. Haskell, 51. New York: R. R. Bowker Co., 1979.
33 Bruce Arneill, and Karrie Frasca-Beaulieu, "Healing Environments: Architecture and Design Conducive to Health." In *Putting Patients First: Designing and Practicing Patient-centered Care*, edited by Susan B. Frampton, Laura Gilpin, and Patrick A. Charmel, 166. San Francisco, CA: Jossey-Bass, 2003.
34 American Hospital Association, *Signs and Graphics*, 7–9.
35 Lynch, Kevin, and Gary Hack. *Site planning*, 3rd ed. Cambridge, MA: The MIT Press, 1984.
36 The Center for Universal Design. "About Universal Design." The Center for Universal Design, 2008. http://www.ncsu.edu/ncsu/design/cud/about_ud/about_ud.htm
37 See, for example: Cooper Marcus, Clare, and Marni Barnes (Eds). *Healing Gardens: Therapeutic Benefits and Design Recommendations*. New York: Wiley, 1999; Gesler, Wilbert M. *Healing Places*. New York: Rowman & Littlefield Publishers, Inc., 2003.
38 Kaplan, Rachel, Stephen Kaplan, and Terry Brown. "Environmental Preference: A Comparison of Four Domains of Predictors." *Environment and Behavior 21*, (1989): 509–530. doi:10.1177/0013916589215001
39 Ulrich, Roger S. "View Through a Window May Enhance Recovery from Surgery." *Science* 224(4647), (1984, April 27): 420–421.

40 Kaplan, Kaplan, and Brown. "Environmental Preference," 524.
41 Herzog, Thomas. "A Cognitive Analysis of Preference for Waterscapes." *Journal of Environmental Psychology* 5, (1985): 225–241. doi:10.1016/S0272-4944(85)80024-4
42 Buhyoff, Gregory J., and John D. Wellman. "Seasonality Bias in Landscape Preference Research," *Leisure Sciences* 2, (1979): 181–190.
43 Cooper Marcus, and Barnes. *Healing Gardens: Therapeutic Benefits and Design Recommendations.*
44 Clare Cooper Marcus, and Marni Barnes, "Introduction: Historic and Cultural Overview." In *Healing Gardens: Therapeutic Benefits and Design Recommendations,* edited by Clare Cooper Marcus and Marni Barnes, 4. New York: John Wiley & Sons, Inc., 1999.
45 Cooper Marcus, Clare, and Marni Barnes. *Gardens in Health Care Facilities: Uses, Therapeutic Benefits, and Design Considerations.* Martinez, CA: Center for Health Design, 1995; Francis, Carolyn, and Clare Cooper Marcus. "Restorative Places: Environment and Emotional Well-Being." In *Proceedings of the 23rd Environmental Design Research Association Conference*, edited by Ernesto G. Arias and Mark D. Gross, 274. Oklahoma City, OK: EDRA, 1992.
46 Whitehouse, Sandra, James W. Vanai, Michael Seid, Clare Cooper Marcus, Mary Jane Ensberg, Jennifer R. Jacobs, and Robyn S. Mehlenbeck. "Evaluating a Children's Hospital Garden Environment: Utilization and Consumer Satisfaction." *Journal of Environmental Psychology* 21(3), (2001): 301–314. See also research cited in Carpman, Grant, and Simmons. *Design that Cares: Planning Health Facilities for Patients and Visitors.*
47 Ulrich, Roger S. "Effects of Gardens on Health Outcomes: Theory and Research." In *Healing Gardens: Therapeutic Benefits and Design Recommendations,* edited by Clare Cooper Marcus and Marni Barnes, 27–86; 36. New York: John Wiley & Sons, Inc., 1999.
48 Cooper Marcus, and Barnes, *Gardens in Healthcare Facilities: Uses, Therapeutic Benefits, and Design Recommendations.*
49 Ulrich, "Effects of Gardens on Health Outcomes: Theory and Research."
50 Cooper Marcus, Clare, and Marni Barnes, "Design Philosophy." In *Healing Gardens: Therapeutic Benefits and Design Recommendations,* edited by Clare Cooper Marcus, and Marni Barnes, 91. New York: John Wiley & Sons, Inc., 1999.
51 Cooper Marcus, Clare, and Marni Barnes, "Acute Care General Hospitals: Case Studies and Design Guidelines." In *Healing Gardens: Therapeutic Benefits and Design Recommendations,* edited by Clare Cooper Marcus and Marni Barnes, 212. New York: John Wiley & Sons, Inc., 1999.
52 Cooper Marcus, and Barnes, "Acute Care General Hospitals: Case Studies and Design Guidelines," 197–214.
53 Carpman, Grant, and Simmons, *Design that Cares,* 202.
54 Cooper Marcus, and Barnes, "Acute Care General Hospitals: Case Studies and Design Guidelines," 228.
55 Carpman, Grant, and Simmons, *Design that Cares,* 208
56 Cooper Marcus, and Barnes, "Acute Care General Hospitals: Case Studies and Design Guidelines," 213.

Chapter 2

1 Street, Richard L., Jr. "Information-giving in Medical Consultations: The Influence of Patients' Communication Styles and Personal Characteristics." *Social Science & Medicine* 32(5), (1991): 541–548. doi:10.1016/0277-9536(91)90288-N
2 Lowrey, Annie, and Robert Pear. "Doctor Shortage Likely to Worsen with Health Law. Primary Care is Scarce." *The New York Times*, July 28, 2012. http://www.nytimes.com/2012/07/29/health/policy/too-few-doctors-in-many-us-communities.html?_r=0
3 Leather, Phil, Diane Beale, Angeli Santos, Janine Watts, and Laura Lee. "Outcomes of Environmental Appraisal of Different Hospital Waiting Areas." *Environment and Behavior* 35(6), (2003): 842–869. doi:10.1177/0013916503254777

Notes

4. Mattera, Marianne. "Doctors Like Books are Judged by Their Covers – Like It or Not." *MedPageToday*, January 7, 2010, Para. 9. http://www.medpagetoday.com/Blogs/InOtherWords/17846
5. Becker, Franklin, and Stephanie Douglass. "The Ecology of the Patient Visit: Physical Attractiveness, Waiting Times, and Perceived Quality of Care." *Journal of Ambulatory Care Management* 31(2), (2008): 128–141. doi:10.1097/01.JAC.0000314703.34795.44
6. Arneill, Allison B., and Ann Sloan Devlin. "Perceived Quality of Care: The Influence of the Waiting Room Environment" (see chap. 1, n. 9).
7. Becker and Douglass, *The Ecology of the Patient Visit*, 137.
8. Lowes, Robert. "Starting a Practice 5–6 months Out: Office Design and Supplies." *Modern Medicine*, June 18, 2004. http://www.modernmedicine.com/modernmedicine/article/articleDetail.jsp?id=108968
9. Newman, Oscar. *Defensible Space: Crime Prevention through Urban Design*. New York: Macmillan, 1973.
10. Weverka, Peter. "Plan a Medical Office Layout." Office.Microsoft.com. Accessed August 1, 2013. http://office.microsoft.com/en-us/visio-help/plan-a-medical-office-layout-HA001189434.aspx
11. O'Brien, Dennis. Maps and Wayfinding, LLC, in an e-mail message to the author, September 9, 2013.
12. Moeser, Shannon Dawn. "Cognitive Mapping in a Complex Building." *Environment and Behavior* 20(1), (1988): 21–49. doi:10.1177/0013916588201002
13. Weisman, Gerald D. "Evaluating Architectural Legibility: Way-Finding in the Built Environment. *Environment and Behavior* 13(2), (1981): 189–204. doi:10.1177/0013916581132004
14. Weisman, Gerald D. "Improving Wayfinding and Architectural Legibility in Housing for the Elderly," (see chap. 1, n. 25).
15. Weisman, "Improving Wayfinding and Architectural Legibility in Housing for the Elderly," 456.
16. Guglielmo, Wayne J. "Re-engineering Your Practice: Make Your Office Layout Serves Your Needs." *Modern Medicine*, June 19, 2000. http://www.modernmedicine.com/modernmedicine/article/articleDetail.jsp?id=121232
17. Malkin, Jain. *Medical and Dental Space Planning: A Comprehensive Guide to Design, Equipment, and Clinical Procedures*, 3rd ed. New York: John Wiley & Sons, Inc., 2002, 32–34.
18. Connected Technology Solutions. "Patient Passport Express™." Connected Technology Solutions. Accessed August 1, 2013. http://www.connectedts.com/interactive-kiosk/by-customer/patient-passport-express/
19. Horowitz, Brian T. "CTS, Phreesia Self-Service Units Replace Medical Office Check-in Paperwork." eWeek. January 28, 2011, Para. 5. http://www.eweek.com/c/a/Health-Care-IT/CTS-Phreesia-SelfService-Units-Replace-Medical-Office-CheckIn-Paperwork-745330/,
20. Herczeg, Laszlo. "It's Not Just about Time: A Fuelfor Design Exploration into the Experience of Waiting in Heathcare." Barcelona: Fuelfor, 2011, p. 49 http://issuu.com/fuelfor/docs/waitbook_pdf/8?e 326 4945/3977126
21. Alderman, Lesley. "The Doctor Will See You…Eventually." *The New York Times*, August 1, 2011. http://www.nytimes.com/2011/08/02/health/policy/02consumer.html?_r=1&pagewanted=print
22. Press Ganey. "Medical Practice Top Improvers – A Client Resource of Innovation and Best Practices." Press Ganey, 2007. http://www.pressganey.com/newslanding/10-09-20/Medical_Practice_Top_Improvers_-_A_Resource_of_Innovations_and_Best_Practices.aspx
23. Press Ganey, "Medical Practice Top Improvers," 5.
24. Altman, *The Environment and Social Behavior*, 18, (see Introduction, n. 23).
25. Altman, *The Environment and Social Behavior*, 11.
26. Langer, Ellen J., and Judith Rodin. "The Effects of Choice and Enhanced Personal Responsibility for the Aged: A Field Experiment in an Institutional Setting." *Journal of Personality and Social Psychology* 34(2), (1976): 191–198. doi:10.1037/0022-3514.34.2.191
27. Hall, Edward T. *The Hidden Dimension*. Garden City, New York: Anchor Books, Double & Company, Inc., 1969.

28 Felipe, Nancy Jo, and Robert Sommer. "Invasions of Personal Space." *Social Problems* 14, (1966): 206–214.
29 Hall, *The Hidden Dimension*, 117–119.
30 Pennachio, Dorothy L. "Practice Pointers. Your Waiting Room: Creat a First-rate Impression." *Medical Economics*, November 7, 2003. http://medicaleconomics.modernmedicine.com/medical-economics/news/practice-pointersyour-waiting-room-create-first-rate-impression
31 Holahan, Charles. "Seating Patterns and Patient Behavior in an Experimental Dayroom." *Journal of Abnormal Psychology* 80(2), (1972): 115–124.
32 Bergersen, Cindy Lee. "Furniture Arrangement Part 1: Creating Conversation Areas Worth Talking About." Hamptons.com. June 18, 2008. http://www.hamptons.com/Lifestyle//Garden-And-Interior-Design/4081/Furniture-Arrangement-Part-I-Creating.html?articleID=4081#.Ud1r--CAatE
33 Pennachio, "Practice Pointers."
34 Labaree, Suzanne. "Six Ways to Improve Doctors' Waiting Rooms." Co.Design: business + innovation + design. August 16, 2011. http://www.fastcodesign.com/1664797/six-ways-to-improve-doctors-waiting-rooms
35 Becker and Douglass, "The Ecology of the Patient Visit," 139–140.
36 Sommer, Robert. *Tight Spaces: Hard Architecture and How to Humanize It.* Englewood Cliffs, NJ: Prentice Hall, 1974.
37 Lowes, "Starting a Practice 5–6 Months Out: Office Design and Supplies."
38 Malkin, "*Medical and Dental Space Planning*, 332; see also 31.
39 Pennachio, "Practice Pointers."
40 White, Robert W. "Motivation Reconsidered: The Concept of Competence," (see Introduction, n. 21).
41 Herczeg, "It's Not Just About Time.
42 Becker and Douglass, "The Ecology of the Patient Visit," 134–135.
43 Lee, So Young, and Jay L. Brand. "Effects of Control Over Office Workspace on Perceptions of the Work Environment and Work Outcomes." *Journal of Environmental Psychology* 25(3), (2005): 323–333. doi:10.1016/j.jenvp.2005.08.001
44 Ulrich, Roger S. "Effects of Interior Design on Wellness: Theory and Recent Scientific Research." *Journal of Health Care Interior Design* 3, (1991): 97–109.
45 Reuters. "More Than Half of Americans Use Internet for Health," (see Introduction, n. 18).
46 Mills, Peter R., Susannah Tomkins, and Luc J. M. Schlangen. "The Effect of High Correlated Colour Temperature Office Lighting on Employee Wellbeing and Work Performance." *Journal of Circadian Rhythms* 5(2) (2007). doi:10.1186/1740-3391-5-2
47 Walch, Jeffrey M., Bruce S. Rabin, Richard Day, Jessica N. Williams, Krissy Choi, and James D. Kang. "The Effect of Sunlight on Post-operative Analgesic Medication Usage: A Prospective Study of Patients Undergoing Spinal Surgery." *Psychosomatic Medicine* 67(1), (2005): 156–163.
48 Malone, Eileen B., and Barbara A. Dellinger. "Furniture Design Features and Healthcare Outcomes." Center for Health Design, May 2011. http://www.healthdesign.org/chd/research/furniture-design-features-and-healthcare-outcomes
49 Malkin, *Medical and Dental Space Planning*, 533–540; upholstery 543–544.
50 Nemschoff. "Products." Nemschoff. Accessed December 10, 2013. http://www.nemschoff.com/products/categories/lounge-seating
51 Nemschoff. "Nemschoff Performance Fabrics." Nemschoff. Accessed December 10, 2013. http://www.nemschoff.com/design-resources/materials/fabrics
52 Nurture® by Steelcase. "High Functioning Waiting Environments." Nurture® by Steelcase. Accessed December 10, 2013. http://www.nurture.com/applications/waiting-areas/
53 Nurture® by Steelcase. "High Functioning Waiting Environments."
54 Steelcase. "Case Study. Mayo Clinic. SPARC Innovation Program." Steelcase, 2012. http://www.nurture.com/wp-content/uploads/2012/04/Mayo-Clinic-Case-Study.pdf
55 Malkin, *Medical and Dental Space Planning*, 61.
56 Malkin, *Medical and Dental Space Planning*, 64.

Notes

57 Puffer, Bruce. "Design for a New Medical Office." *Physician's News Digest,* February 20, 1997. http://www.physiciansnews.com/1997/02/20/design-for-a-new-medical-office/
58 Karro, Jonathan, Andrew W. Dent, and Stephen Farish. "Patient Perceptions of Privacy Infringements in an Emergency Department." *Emergency Medicine Australasia* 17(2), (2003): 117–123. doi:10.1111/j.1742-6723.2005.00702.x
59 Hagerman, Inger, Gundars Rasmanis, Vanja Blomkvist, Roger Ulrich, Claire Anne Eriksen, and Töres Theorell. "Influence of Intensive Coronary Care Acoustics on the Quality of Care and Physiological State of Patients." *International Journal of Cardiology* 98(2), (2005): 267–270.
60 Hamilton, D. Kirk, and Mardelle McCuskey Shepley. *Design for Critical Care: An Evidence-Based Approach*. New York: Architectural Press, 2010.
61 Hamilton and Shepley, *Design for Critical Care*, 138.
62 Malkin, *Medical and Dental Space Planning*, 364.
63 Malkin, *Medical and Dental Space Planning*, 67.
64 Malkin, *Medical and Dental Space Planning*, 308.
65 Malkin, *Medical and Dental Space Planning*, 66.
66 Kira, Alexander. *The Bathroom*. New York: The Viking Press, 1976, 107.
67 Kira, *The Bathroom*, 165.
68 Malkin, Jain. *A Visual Reference for Evidence-Based Design*. Concord, CA: The Center for Health Design, 2008, 126.
69 Kira, *The Bathroom*, 212.
70 Hamilton and Shepley, *Design for Critical Care,* 138.
71 Malkin, *Medical and Dental Space Planning*, 36, 90.
72 Malkin, *Medical and Dental Space Planning*, 115.
73 Kira, *The Bathroom*, 211.
74 Malkin, *Medical and Dental Space Planning*, 115.
75 Redway, Keith, and Shameem Fawdar. "A Comparative Study of Three Different Hand Drying Methods: Paper Towel, Warm Air Dryer, Jet Dryer. *European Tissue Symposium*. London: University of Westminster, November 2008. http://www.europeantissue.com/pdfs/090402-2008%20WUS%20Westminster%20University%20hygiene%20study,%20nov2008.pdf
76 Malkin, *A Visual Reference*, 126.
77 Malkin, *A Visual Reference*, 7.64; 7.65.

Chapter 3

1 McGill, Doug. "Devola Funk's Health Care Reminder: 'You Feel Healthier When You're Dressed.'" November 23, 2010. http://blog.centerforinnovation.mayo.edu/discussion/devola-funks-health-care-reminder-you-feel-healthier-when-youre-dressed
2 Seligman, Martin E., Steven F. Maier, and James H. Geer. "Alleviation of Learned Helplessness in the Dog." *Journal of Abnormal Psychology* 73(3), (1968): 256–262.
3 Kessels, Roy P. C. "Patients' Memory for Medical Information." *Journal of the Royal Society of Medicine* 96(5), (2003): 219–222. doi:10.1258/jrsm.96.5.219
4 Ley, Philip. "Memory for Medical Information." *British Journal of Social and Clinical Psychology* 18(2), (1979): 245–255. doi:10.1111/j.2044-8260.1979.tb00333.x
5 Watson, Philip W. B., and Brian McKinstry. "A Systematic Review of Interventions to Improve Recall of Medical Advice in Healthcare Consultations." *Journal of the Royal Society of Medicine* 102(6), (2009): 235–243. doi:10.1258/jrsm.2009.090013
6 Cahnman, Sheila F. "Outpatient Options: A Look at the Changing Ambulatory Care Facility." *Health Facilities Management*. June, 2011. http://www.hfmmagazine.com/hfmmagazine/jsp/articledisplay.jsp?dcrpath=HFMMAGAZINE/Article/data/06JUN2011/0611HFM_FEA_AD&domain=HFMMAGAZINE

7. Almquist, Julka, Caroline Kelly, and Joyce Bromberg. "The Relationship Between Workspace, Activity and Hierarchy in a Clinical Exam Room: An Innovative Design in Practice." Presentation at the 39th Annual Conference of the Environmental Design Research Association, Veracruz, Mexico, May, 2008.
8. Almquist, Julka R., Caroline Kelly, Joyce Bromberg, Sandra C. Bryant, Teresa J. H. Christianson, and Victor M. Montori. "Consultation Room Design and the Clinical Encounter: The Space and Interaction Randomized Trial." *Health Environments Research & Design Journal* 3(1), (2009): 41–78.
9. Mayo Clinic. Center for Innovation. "Design Thinking." Mayo Clinic. Center for Innovation. Accessed December 10, 2013. http://www.mayo.edu/center-for-innovation/what-we-do/design-thinking
10. Manning, Harley, and Kerry Bodine. *Outside In: The Power of Putting Customers at the Center of Your Business.* New York: New Harvest, Houghton Mifflin Harcourt, 2012.
11. Calandra, Robert. "Redesigning an Office? Opt for Simplicity and Comfort." *ACP Internist*®, 2. July-August, 2005, para. 22. http://www.acpinternist.org/archives/2005/07/design.htm
12. Calandra, "Redesigning an Office?".
13. Agency for Healthcare Research and Quality. *Making Health Care Safer: A Critical Analysis of Patient Safety Practices.* Rockville, MD: AHRQ, 2001.
14. HermanMiller Healthcare. "Patient-Room Design: The Same-Handed, Mirror Image Debate. Research Summary." HermanMiller Healthcare, 2011. http://www.hermanmiller.com/MarketFacingTech/hmc/research/research_summaries/assets/wp_Same_vs_Mirror.pdf
15. Watkins, Nicholas W., Mary M. Kennedy, Maria M. Ducharme, and Cynthia C. Padula. "Same-handed and Mirrored Unit Configurations: Is There a Difference in Patient and Nurse Outcomes?" *Journal of Nursing Administration* 41(6), (2011): 273–279. doi:10.1097/NNA.0b013e31821c47b4
16. Stichler, Jaynelle F., and Cindi McCullough. "Same-handed Patient Room Configurations: Anecdotal and Empirical Evidence." *Journal of Nursing Administration* 42(3), (2012): 125–130. doi.10.1097/NNA.0b013e318248073d
17. Winograd, Eugene, and Robert M. Soloway. "On Forgetting the Locations of Things Stored in Special Places." *Journal of Experimental Psychology: General* 115(4), (1986): 366–372. doi:10.1037/0096-3445.115.4.366
18. HermanMiller Healthcare, "Patient-Room Design," 5.
19. Microsoft Office. "Medical Office Layout." Microsoft Office. Accessed December 10, 2013. http://office.microsoft.com/en-us/templates/medical-office-layout-TC001194549.aspx
20. Calandra, "Redesigning an Office?".
21. Cahnman, "Outpatient Options," 4.
22. Davignon, Keith, Vision 3 Architects, e-mail exchange with the author, September 4, 2013.
23. Malkin, Jain. "Evidence-Based Design that Reflects Patient-Centered Care: A Journey from Father Knows Best to Have It Your Way." Part of the Intensive: Implementing Person-Centered Design in Healthcare: Building Connections at the 42nd annual Environmental Design Research Association Conference, Chicago, Illinois, May 2011.
24. Cahnman, "Outpatient Options," 6.
25. Kupritz, Virginia W., and Teresa A. Bellingar, "Quantitative Assessment of Individual and Group Privacy Needs." In *Building Sustainable Communities: Proceedings of the 38th Annual Environmental Design Research Association Conference*, edited by Janice M. Bissell, 208. Edmond, OK: EDRA, 2007.
26. Casciato, Daniel. "Soundproofing Your Office." *Medical Office Today*, August 17, 2010. http://www.medicalofficetoday.com/article/soundproofing-your-office
27. Olsen, Jon C., and Brad R. Sabin. "Emergency Department Patient Perceptions of Privacy and Confidentiality." *Journal of Emergency Medicine* 25(3), (2003): 329–333. doi:10.1016/S0736-4679(03)00216-6
28. Joseph, Anjali, and Roger Ulrich. "Sound Control for Improved Outcomes in Healthcare Settings." Issue Paper 4. The Center for Health Design. January, 2007. http://www.healthdesign.org/sites/default/files/Sound%20Control.pdf
29. Joseph and Ulrich, "Sound Control," 7.

Notes

30 HermanMiller Healthcare. "Sound Practices: Noise Control in the Health Environment. Research Summary," HermanMiller Healthcare. 2006. http://www.hermanmiller.com/research/research-summaries/sound-practices-noise-control-in-the-healthcare-environment.html
31 HermanMiller Healthcare, "Sound Practices, 6–7.
32 Deshefy-Longhi, Terry, Jane Karpe Dixon, Douglas Olsen, and Margaret Grey. "Privacy and Confidentiality Issues in Primary Care: Views of Advanced Practice Nurses and Their Patients." *Nursing Ethics* 11(4), (2004): 378–393. doi:10.1191/0969733004ne710oa
33 Deshefy-Longhi, *et al.*, "Privacy and Confidentiality," 391–392.
34 Casciato, "Soundproofing Your Office," 3.
35 Weidman, Ted. "Psychologist Office Sound Problem." Acoustical Surfaces-Soundproofing Blog, July 24, 2008. http://www.acousticalsurfaces.com/blog/soundproofing/psychologist-office-sound-problem/
36 Office for Civil Rights. *Incidental Uses and Disclosures [45 CFR 164.502 (a) (1) (iii)]*. OCR HIPAA Privacy, December 3, 2002. http://www.hhs.gov/ocr/privacy/hipaa/understanding/coveredentities/incidentalu&d.pdf
37 Hongisto, Valtteri, Annu Haapakangas, and Miia Haka. "Task Performance and Speech Intelligibility – A Model to Promote Noise Control Actions in Open Offices." *Performance: 9th International Congress on Noise as a Public Health Problem (ICBEN)*, 2008. http://www.icben.org/2008/PDFs/Hongisto_et_al.pdf
38 Green Guide for Health Care™. *Acoustic Environment Technical Brief*. Green Guide for Health Care™. Version 2.2, 2007. http://www.gghc.org/documents/TechBriefs/GGHC_TechBrief_Acoustic-Environment.pdf.
39 Hilton, B. Ann. "Noise in Acute Patient Care Areas." *Research in Nursing & Health* 8(3), (1985): 283–291.
40 Bayo, Maria V., Ana M. Garcia, and Amando Garcia. "Noise Levels in an Urban Hospital and Workers' Subjective Responses." *Archives of Environmental Health* 50(3), (1995): 247–251.
41 Malkin, *Medical and Dental Space Planning*, 558 (see chap. 2, n. 17).
42 Koriwchak, Mike. "Build EMR Functionality Into the Exam Room." *Kevin MD.com*. February 9, 2011. http://www.kevinmd.com/blog/2011/02/build-emr-functionality-exam-room.html
43 Shachak, Aviv, and Shmuel Reis. "The Impact of Electronic Medical Records on Patient-Doctor Communication During Consultation: A Narrative Literature Review." *Journal of Evaluation in Clinical Practice* 15(4), (2009): 641–649. doi:10.1111/j.1365-2753.2008.01065.x
44 Rouf, Emran, Heidi S. Chumley, and Alison E. Dobbie. "Electronic Health Records in Outpatient Clinics." *BMC Medical Education* 8(13), (2008): 1–7. doi:10.1186/1472-6920-8-13. http://www.biomedcentral.com/content/pdf/1472-6920-8-13.pdf
45 Booth, Nick, Paul Robinson, and Judy Kohannejad. "Identification of High-Quality Consultation Practice in Primary Care: The Effects of Computer Use on Doctor-Patient Rapport." *Informatics in Primary Care* 12(2), (2004): 75–83.
46 Holzinger, Andreas, Markus Baernthaler, Walter Pammer, Herman Katz, Vesna Bjelic-Radisic, and Martina Ziefle. "Investigating Paper vs. Screen in Real-Life Hospital Workflows: Performance Contradicts Perceived Superiority of Paper in the User Experience." *International Journal of Human-Computer Studies* 69(9), (2011): 563–570. doi:10.1016/j.ijhes.2011.05.002
47 Frankel, Richard, Andrea Altschuler, Sheba George, James Kinsman, Holly Jimison, Nan R. Robertson, and John Hsu. "Effects of Exam-Room Computing on Clinician-Patient Communication: A Longitudinal Qualitative Study." *Journal of General Internal Medicine* 20(8), (2005): 677–682. doi:10.1111/j.1525-1497.2005.0163.x, 681.
48 Calandra, "Redesigning an Office?".
49 Shachak and Reis, "The Impact of Electronic Medical Records," 645.
50 Beck, Rainer S., Rebecca Daughtridge, and Philip D. Sloane. "Physician-Patient Communication in the Primary Care Office. A Systematic Review." *Journal of the American Board of Family Practice* 15(1), (2002): 25–38.

51 Miwa, Yoshiko, and Kaxunori Hanyu. "The Effect of Interior Design on Communication and Impressions of a Counselor in a Counseling Room." *Environment and Behavior* 38(4), (2006): 484–502. doi:10.1177/001391650528084

52 Flynn, John E. *Architectural Interior Systems: Lighting, Acoustics, and Air Conditioning,* 3rd ed. New York: Van Nostrand Reinhold, 1992.

53 Arneill and Frasca-Beaulieu, "Healing Environments," 185, (see chap. 1, n. 33).

54 Benya, James R. "Lighting for Healing." *Journal of Health Care Interior Design* 1, (1989): 55–58.

55 Benya, "Lighting for Healing," 57.

56 Benya, "Lighting for Healing," 58.

57 Choi, Joon-Ho, Liliana O. Beltran, and Hway-Suh Kim. "Impacts of Indoor Daylight Environments on Patient Average Length of Stay (ALOS) in a Healthcare Facility." *Building and Environment* 50, (2012): 65–75. doi:10.1016/j.buildenv.2011.10.01

58 Choi, Beltran, and Kim, "Impacts of Indoor Daylight Environments," 74.

59 The Green Economy. "Study Shows Significant Improvement of School Results With Philips Dynamic Lighting Classroom System." The Green Economy. May 28, 2010. http://www.thegreeneconomy.com/study-shows-significant-improvement-of-school-results-with-philips-dynamic-lighting-classroom-system/

60 Smolders, Karin C. H. J., Yvonne A. W. De Kort, and Pierre J. M. Cluitmans. "A Higher Illuminance Induces Alertness Even During Office Hours: Findings on Subjective Measures, Task Performance and Heart Rate Measures." *Physiology & Behavior* 107(1), (2012): 7–16. doi:10.1016/jphysbeh.2012.04.028

61 Calandra, "Redesigning an Office?" 3.

62 Graf Klein, Judy. *The Office Book: Ideas and Designs for Contemporary Work Spaces.* New York: Facts on File, Inc., 1982, 20.

63 Wells, Meredith, and Luke Thelen. "What Does Your Workspace Say About You? The Influence of Personality, Status, and Workspace on Personalization." *Environment and Behavior* 34(3), (2002): 300–321. doi:10.1177/0013916502034003002

64 Devlin, Ann Sloan, Sarah Donovan, Arianne Nicolov, Olivia Nold, Andrea Packard, and Gabrielle Zandan. "'Impressive?' Credentials, Family Photographs, and the Perception of Therapist Qualities." *Journal of Environmental Psychology* 29(4), (2009): 503–512. doi:10.1016/j.envp.2009.08.008

65 Gosling, Samuel D., Sei Jin Ko, Thomas Mannarelli, and Margaret E. Morris, "A Room with a Cue: Personality Judgments Based on Offices and Bedrooms." *Journal of Personality and Social Psychology* 82(3), (2002): 379–398.

66 Wahl, Otto, and Eli Aroesty-Cohen. "Attitudes of Mental Health Professionals About Mental Illness: A Review of the Recent Literature." *Journal of Community Psychology* 38(1), (2010): 49–62. doi:10.1002/jcop.20351

67 Hoffman, Jan. "When Your Therapist Is Only a Click Away." *The New York Times*, September 23, 2011. http://www.nytimes.com/2011/09/25/fashion/therapists-are-seeing-patients-online.html?pagewanted=all&_r=0

68 Simpson, Susan. "Psychotherapy Via Videoconferencing: A Review." *British Journal of Guidance & Counselling* 37(3), (2009): 271–286. doi:10.1080/03069880902957007

69 Newhill, Christina E. "Risk Assessment, Violent Clients and Practitioner Safety: Workshop Handout" SocialWorkPodcast.com. Accessed August 1, 2013. http://www.socialworkpodcast.com/Client%20Violence%20Workshop%20Handout.pdf

70 See for example: Devlin, Ann Sloan, Briana Borenstein, Christina Finch, Maurifa Hassan, Erin Iannotti, and Justin Koufopoulos. "Multicultural Art in the Therapy Office: Community and Student Perceptions of the Therapist." *Professional Psychology: Research and Practice* 44(3), (2013): 168–176. doi:10.1037/a0031925; Devlin *et al.* "'Impressive?' Credentials, Family Photographs, and the Perception of Therapist Qualities,"; Devlin, Ann Sloan, and Jack L. Nasar. "Impressions of Psychotherapists' Offices: Do Therapists and Clients Agree?" *Professional Psychology: Research and Practice* 43(2), (2012): 118–122. doi:10.1037/a0027292; Nasar, Jack L. and Ann Sloan Devlin. "Impressions of Psychotherapists' Offices." *Journal of Counseling Psychology* 58(3), (2011): 310–320.

Notes

doi:10.1037/a00238872011; Devlin, Ann Sloan, Jack L. Nasar, and Ebru Cubukcu. "Students' Impressions of Psychotherapists' Offices: Cross-Cultural Comparisons." *Environment and Behavior*. Advance Online publication, August 22, 2013. doi:10.1177/0013916513498602

71 Devlin *et al*., "'Impressive?' Credentials, Family Photographs, and the Perception of Therapist Qualities."
72 Green, Penelope. "What's in a Chair?" *The New York Times*, March 6, 2008. http://www.nytimes.com/2008/03/06/garden/06shrink.html
73 Nasar and Devlin, "Impressions of Psychotherapists' Offices."
74 Devlin and Nasar, "Impressions of Psychotherapists' Offices: Do Therapists and Clients Agree?"
75 Devlin, Nasar, and Cubukcu, "Students' Impressions of Psychotherapists' Offices: Cross-Cultural Comparisons."
76 Mathews, *How to Succeed*, 39, (see Introduction, n. 4).
77 Mathews, *How to Succeed*, 39.
78 *The Office Practitioner*, "Advice to Young Doctors – Opening and Furnishing an Office." *The Office Practitioner* 2(7), (1905): 149–150.
79 *The Office Practitioner*, "Advice to Young Doctors," 149.
80 Davis, *History of Harrison County*, 504, (see chap. 1, n. 6).
81 Davis, *History of Harrison County*, 505.
82 *The Office Practitioner*, "How to Conduct Your Office." *The Office Practitioner*, 2(11), (1905): 225.
83 Davis, *History of Harrison County*, 500.
84 Mathews, *How to Succeed*, 40.
85 Cathell, *The Physician Himself,* 11, (see Introduction, n. 1).
86 *The Office Practitioner*, "Advice to Young Doctors – Opening and Furnishing an Office."

Chapter 4

1 Catania, Chiara, T. De Pas, I. Michella, F. DeBraud, D. Micheli, L. Adamoli, G. Spitaleri, C. Noberasco, A. Milani, M. G. Zampino, F. Toffalorio, D. Radice, A Goldhirsch, and F. Nolè, "Waiting and the Waiting Room: How do You Experience Them? Emotional Implications and Suggestions from Patients with Cancer." *Journal of Cancer Education* 26, (2011): 393.
2 Arneill and Frasca-Beaulieu, "Healing Environments," 181–182, (see chap. 1, n. 33).
3 Leather, *et al*. "Outcomes of Environmental Appraisal of Different Hospital Waiting Areas," (see chap. 2, n. 3).
4 Ingham, B., and Christopher Spencer. "Do Comfortable Chairs and Soft Light in the Waiting Area Really Help Reduce Anxiety and Improve the Practice's Image?" *Health Psychology Update* 28, (1997): 17–20.
5 Anderson, John R., *Cognitive Psychology and Its Implications*, 7th ed. New York: Worth Publishers, 2010, 32.
6 Anderson, *Cognitive Psychology*, 70.
7 Henderson, John M. "Human Gaze Control During Real-World Scene Perception." *TRENDS in Cognitive Science* 7(11), (2003): 498–504. doi:10.1016/j.tics.2003.09.006
8 Hamid, Sahar N., Brian Stankiewicz, and Mary Hayhoe. "Gaze patterns in Navigation: Encoding Information in Large-Scale Environments." *Journal of Vision* 10(12), (2010): 1–11. doi:10.1167/10.12.28
9 ADAAG. "4.30.6 Signage: Mounting Location and Height." *ADA Accessibility Guidelines for Buildings and Facilities*, September, 2002. http://www.access-board.gov/guidelines-and-standards/buildings-and-sites/about-the-ada-standards/background/adaag
10 Ulrich, Roger S., Robert F. Simons, and Mark A. Miles, "Effects of Environmental Simulations and Television on Blood Donor Stress," *Journal of Architectural and Planning Research* 20(1), (2003): 41.
11 Ulrich, Simons, and Miles, "Effects of Environmental Simulations," 45.
12 Arneill and Frasca-Beaulieu, "Healing Environments," 174.

13. Mazer, Susan, and Dallas Smith, *Sound Choices: Using Music to Design the Environments in Which You Live, Work, and Heal*. Carlsbad, CA: Hay House, Inc., 1999, 157–158.
14. Pruyn, Ad, and Ale Smidts. "Effects of Waiting on the Satisfaction with the Service: Beyond Objective Time Measures." *International Journal of Research in Marketing* 15(4), (1998): 321–334. doi:10.1016/S0167-8116(98)00008-1
15. Hamilton, Melissa M. "Healing Can Begin in Your Waiting Room." *Modern Medicine*, May 10, 2011. http://www.modernmedicine.com/modernmedicine/article/articleDetail.jsp?id=722652
16. Gaerig, Chris. "Televisions in Waiting Rooms," *Healthcare Design* June 15, 2010, para. 5. http://www.healthcaredesignmagazine.com/blogs/cgaerig/televisions-waiting-rooms
17. Pruyn and Smidts, "Effects of Waiting," 321.
18. Tsai, Chun-Yen, Mu-Chia Wang, Wei-Tsen Liao, Jui-Heng Lu, Pi-hung Sun, Blossom Yen-Ju Lin, and Gerald-Mark Breen. "Hospital Outpatient Perceptions of the Physical Environment of Waiting Areas: The Role of Patient Characteristics on Atmospherics in One Academic Medical Center." *BMC Health Services Research* 7 (2007): 198–206. doi:10.1186/1472-6963-7-198
19. Mazer, Susan E. "Music and Nature at the Bedside: Part II of a Two-Part Series." *Research Design Connections*, Issue 1, 2010, para. 1. http://researchdesignconnections.com/pub/2010-issue-I/music-and-nature-bedside-part-ii-two-part-series
20. Mazer, Susan E. "Hospital Noise and the Patient Experience: Seven Ways to Create and Maintain a Quieter Environment." HealingHealth.com. 2010. https://www.premierinc.com/safety/safety-share/01-11-downloads/5_Noise.pdf
21. Leemis, Caroline. "ASID: Providing Positive Distractions During the Patient Wait Experience." *Healthcare Design*, June 13, 2010. http://www.healthcaredesignmagazine.com/blogs/acleemis/asid-providing-positive-distractions-during-patient-wait-experience
22. CrockettSTUDIO, "TV's in the Waiting Room? A Design Dilemma," CrockettSTUDIO, March 24, 2011, para. 2. http://crockettstudio.wordpress.com/2011/03/24/tvs-in-the-waiting-room-a-design-dilemma/
23. Katcher, Aaron, Herman Segal, and Aaron T. Beck. "Comparison of Contemplation and Hypnosis for the Reduction of Anxiety and Discomfort During Dental Surgery." *American Journal of Clinical Hypnosis* 27(1), (1984): 14–21. doi:10.1080/00029157.1984.10402583
24. *Aquatic Digest*. "Office Aquariums: An Interview with Dr. Thomas Koonce." *Aquatic Digest*. Accessed August 1, 2013. http://www.aquaticdigest.com/aquarium-articles/office-aquariums-an-interview-with-dr-thomas-koonce/
25. Ulrich, Roger S. "View Through a Window May Influence Recovery from Surgery," (see chap. 1, n. 39); Berman, Marc G., John Jonides, and Stephen Kaplan. "The Cognitive Benefits of Interacting with Nature." *Psychological Science* 19(12), (2008): 1207–1212. doi:10.1111/j.1467-9280.2008.02225.x
26. Malenbaum, Sara, Francis J. Keefe, Amanda C. Williams, Roger Ulrich, and Tarmar J. Sommers. "Pain in Its Environmental Context: Implications for Designing Environments to Enhance Pain Control." *Pain* 134(3), (2008): 241–244. doi:10.1016/j.pain.2007.12.002
27. Gum, Dawn A., AIA, IIDA, Managing Partner, Interior Architecture & Design, PLLC, e-mail message to the author, August 12, 2013.
28. Walch, *et al*. "The Effect of Sunlight on Post-Operative Analgesic Medication Use," (see chap. 2, n. 47).
29. Lowes, Robert. "Starting a Practice 5–6 Months Out: Office Design and Supplies," (see chap. 2, n. 8).
30. Meyers-Levy, Joan, and Rui (Juliet) Zhu. "The Influence of Ceiling Height: The Effect of Priming on the Type of Processing that People Use." *Journal of Consumer Research* 34(2), (2007): 174–186.
31. Keep, Philip J. "Stimulus Deprivation in Windowless Rooms." *Anaesthesia* 32(7), (1977): 598–600.
32. Art Research Institute. "Visual Therapy." Art Research Institute. Accessed August 1, 2013. http://www.visualtherapy.com/index2.php
33. Bringslimark, Tina, Terry Hartig, and Grete Grindal Patil. "Adaptation to Windowlessness: Do Office Workers Compensate for a Lack of Visual Access to the Outdoors?" *Environment and Behavior* 43, (2011): 469–487. doi:10.1177/0013916510368351

34 Heerwagen, Judith H., and Gordon H. Orians. "Adaptations to Windowlessness: A Study of the Use of Visual Décor in Windowed and Windowless Offices." *Environment and Behavior* 18(5), (1986): 623–639. doi:10.1177/00139165861850
35 Shin, Won Sop. "The Influence of Forest View through a Window on Job Satisfaction and Job Stress." *Scandinavian Journal of Forest Research* 22(3), (2007): 248–253. doi:10.1080/02827580701262733
36 Herzog, Thomas R. "A Cognitive Analysis of Preference for Waterscapes," (see chap. 1, n. 41).
37 Ulrich, Roger, and Laura Gilpin. "Healing Arts: Nutrition for the Soul." In *Putting Patients First: Designing and Practicing Patient-Centered Care*, edited by Susan B. Frampton, Laura Gilpin, and Patrick A. Charmel, 117–146. San Francisco, CA: Jossey-Bass, 2003.
38 Robeznieks, Andis. "Design Drought: Water Features Fall Out of Favor Over Germ Concern." Modern Heathcare.com, January 17, 2011. http://www.modernhealthcare.com/article/20110117/MAGAZINE/110119979
39 Kjellgren, Anette, and Hanne Buhrkall. "A Comparison of the Restorative Effect of a Natural Environment with that of a Simulated Natural Environment." *Journal of Environmental Psychology* 30(4), (2010): 464–472. doi:10.1016/j.jenvp.2010.01.011
40 deKort, Yvonne A. W., Anneloes L. Meijnders, A. A. G. Sponselee, and Wijnand A. Ijsselsteijn. "What's Wrong with Virtual Trees? Restoring from Stress in a Mediated Environment." *Journal of Environmental Psychology* 26(4), (2006): 309–320. doi:10.1016/j.jenvp.2006.09.001
41 Beukeboom, Camiel J., Dion Langeveld, and Karin Tanja-Dijkstra. "Stress-Reducing Effects of Real and Artificial Nature in a Hospital Waiting Room." *The Journal of Alternative and Complementary Medicine* 18(4), (2012): 329–333, 332. doi:10.1089/acm.2011.0488
42 Nanda, Upali, H. Lea Barbato Gaydos, Kathy Hathorn, and Nicholas Watkins. "Art and Posttraumatic Stress: A Review of the Literature on the Therapeutic Implications of Artwork for War Veterans with Posttraumatic Stress Disorder." *Environment and Behavior* 42(3), (2010): 376–390. doi:10.1177/0013916510361874; Ulrich, Roger S., Robert F. Simons, Barbara D. Losito, Evelyn Fiorito, Mark A. Miles, and Michael Zelson. "Stress Recovery During Exposure to Natural and Urban Environments." *Journal of Environmental Psychology* 11(3), (1991): 201–230. doi:10.1016/S0272-4944(05)80184-7; Diette, Gregory B., Noah Lechtzin, Edward Haponik, Arline Devrotes, and Haya R. Rubin. "Distraction Therapy with Nature Sights and Sounds Reduces Pain During Flexible Bronchoscopy: A Complementary Approach to Routine Analgesia." *Chest* 123(3), (2003): 941–948. doi:10.1378/chest.123.3.941; Hathorn, Kathy. "The Use of Art in a Health Care Setting." In *Health Care Interior Finishes: Problems and Solutions – An Environmental Services Perspective*, edited by Pamela L. Blyth, 1–11. Washington, DC: American Hospital Assocation, 1993; Ulrich and Gilpin, "Healing Arts"; Miller, Arlene C., L. C. Hickman, and Grace Kawas Lemasters. "A Distraction Technique for Control of Burn Pain." *Journal of Burn Care Rehabilitation* 13(5), (1992): 576–580.
43 Seligmann, Jean, and Laura Buckley. "A Sickroom with a View: A New Artificial Window Brightens Patients' Days." *Newsweek*, March 26, 1990, 61.
44 American Art Resources. "Transforming the Healthcare Experience Through Art." American Art Resources. Accessed August 1, 2013. http://www.americanartresources.com/
45 Cusack, Pearce, Louise Lankston, and Chris Isles. "Impact of Visual Art in Patient Waiting Rooms: Survey of Patients Attending a Transplant Clinic in Dumfries." *Journal of the Royal Society of Medicine Short Reports* 1(6), (2010): 52. doi:10.1258/shorts.2010.010077
46 Eisen, Sarajane L., Roger S. Ulrich, Mardelle M. Shepley, James W. Varni, and Sandra Sherman. "The Stress-Reducing Effects of Art in Pediatric Health Care: Art Preferences of Healthy Children and Hospitalized Children." *Journal of Child Health Care* 12(3), (2008): 173–190. doi:10.1177/1367493508092507
47 Ulrich, "Effects of Gardens on Health Outcomes," (see chap. 1, n. 47).
48 Ulrich and Gilpin, "Healing Arts," 134–136.
49 Hathorn, Kathy, and Upali Nanda. "A Guide to Evidence-Based Art." The Center for Health Design, 2008. http://www.healthdesign.org/sites/default/files/Hathorn_Nanda_Mar08.pdf
50 Hutlock, Todd. "Killing the Visual Noise." *Healthcare Design*, February 24, 2012. http://www.healthcaredesignmagazine.com/blogs/todd-hutlock/killing-visual-noise

51   Arneill and Devlin. "Perceived Quality of Care" (see chap. 1, n. 9).
52   Devlin, Ann Sloan. Unpublished manuscript, 2011.
53   Cathell, *The Physician Himself,* 11 (see Introduction, n. 1).
54   Gosling, *Snoop: What Your Stuff Says About You,* (see Introduction, n. 6).
55   Cathell, *The Physician Himself,* 11.
56   Wood, Nathan Elliott. *Dollars to Doctors, Or, Diplomacy and Prosperity in Medical Practice.* Chicago: The Lion Publishing Company, 1903, 110.
57   Wood, *Dollars to Doctors,* 111.
58   Arneill and Devlin, "Perceived Quality of Care," 357.
59   Mazer, "Music and Nature at the Bedside: Part II of a Two-Part Series"; Mazer, Susan. "Music, Noise, and the Environment of Care: History, Theory, and Practice." *Music and Medicine* 2(3), (2010): 182–191. doi:10.1177/1943862110372773
60   See for example: Thorgaard, Bitten, Birgitte Brønsted Henriksen, Gunhild Pedersbæck, and Inger Thomsen. "Specially Selected Music in the Cardiac Laboratory – An Important Tool for Improvement of Wellbeing of Patients." *European Journal of Cardiovascular Nursing* 3(1), (2004): 21–26. doi:10.1016/j.ejcnurse.2003.10.001; Williamson, Joan W. "The Effects of Ocean Sounds on Sleep After Coronary Artery Bypass Graft Surgery." *American Journal of Critical Care* 1(1), (1992): 91–97.
61   Dileo, Cheryl, and Joke Bradt. *Medical Music Therapy: A Meta-analysis & Agenda for Future Research.* Cherry Hill, NJ: Jeffrey Books, 2005.
62   Cooke, Marie, Wendy Chaboyer, and Mary Anne Hiratos. "Music and Its Effect on Anxiety in Short Waiting Periods: A Critical Appraisal." *Journal of Clinical Nursing* 14(2), (2005): 145–155. doi:10.1111/j.1365-2702.2004.01033.x
63   See Williamson, "The Effects of Ocean Sounds"; Thorgaard *et al.*, "Specially Selected Music"; Ferguson, Eamonn, Ajit Pal Singh, and Nicole A. Cunningham-Snell. "Stress and Blood Donation: Effects of Music and Previous Donation Experience." *British Journal of Psychology* 88(2), (1997): 277–294.
64   McCaffrey, Ruth, and Edward Freeman. "Effect of Music on Chronic Osteoarthritis Pain in Older People." *Journal of Advanced Nursing* 44(5), (2003): 517–524. doi:10.1046/j.0309-2402.2003.02835.x
65   Schorr, Julie A. "Music and Pattern Change in Chronic Pain." *Advances in Nursing Science* 15(4), (1993): 27–36.
66   See, for example: Lee, Daniel W. H., Angus C. W. Chan, Simon K. H. Wong, Terence M. K. Fung, Anthony Chi Ngai Li, Simon K. C. Chan, Lik Man Mui, Ng, K. W. Enders, and Sydney S. C. Chung. "Can Visual Distraction Decrease the Dose of Patient-Controlled Sedation Required During Colonoscopy? A Prospective Randomized Controlled Trial." *Endoscopy* 36(3), (2004): 197–201. doi:10.1055/s-2004-814247; Miller, Hickman, and Lemasters. "A Distraction Technique for Control of Burn Pain."
67   Mazer and Smith, *Sound Choices,* 91.
68   Mazer and Smith, *Sound Choices,* 159.
69   Mazer, Susan E. "Music and Nature at the Bedside: Part One of a Two-Part Series." *Research Design Connections* Issue 4, 2009, Summary, pt. 4. http://researchdesignconnections.com/pub/2009-issue-4/music-and-nature-bedside-part-one-two-part-series
70   Lee, Kwo-Chen, Yuh-Huey Chao, Jia-Jean Yiin, Pei-Yi Chiang, and Yann-Fen Chao. "Effectiveness of Different Music-Playing Devices for Reducing Preoperative Anxiety: A Clinical Control Study." *International Journal of Nursing Studies* 48(10), (2011): 1180–1187. doi:10.1016/j.ijnurstu.2011.04.001
71   Lee, Kwo-Chen, Yuh-Huey Chao, Jia-Jean Yiin, Hsin-Yi Hsieh, Wen-Jan Dai, and Yann-Fen Chao. "Evidence That Music Listening Reduces Preoperative Patients' Anxiety." *Biological Research for Nursing* 14(1), (2012): 78–84. doi:10.1177/1099800410396704
72   Guétin, Stéphane, Patrick Giniès, Didier Kong A. Siou, Marie-Christine Picot, Christelle Pommié, Elisabeth Guldner, Anne-Marie Gosp, Katelyn Ostyn, Emmanuel Coudeyre, and Jacques Touchon.

"The Effects of Music Intervention in the Management of Chronic Pain: A Single-Blind, Randomized, Controlled Trial." *Clinical Journal of Pain* 28, (2012): 329–337. doi:10.1097/AJP.0b013e31822be973
73 The CARE Channel. Resources. http://healinghealth.com/hhs/site/page/articles
74 Mitchell, Laura A., and Raymond A. R. MacDonald. "An Experimental Investigation of the Effects of Preferred and Relaxing Music Listening on Pain Perception." *Journal of Music Therapy* 43(4), (2006): 295–316.
75 Thorgaard et al. "Specially Selected Music."
76 Vaajoki, Anne, Anna-Maija Pietilä, Päivi Kankkunen, and Katri Vehviläinen-Julkunen, "Effects of Listening to Music on Pain Intensity and Pain Distress after Surgery: An Intervention," *Journal of Clinical Nursing* 21(5–6), (2012): 708. doi:10.1111/j.1365-2702.2011.03829.x
77 Arneill and Frasca-Beaulieu, "Healing Environments," 187–188.
78 Leemis, "ASID: Providing Positive Distractions During the Patient Wait Experience."
79 Deitrick, Lynn, Daniel Ray, Glenn Stern, Cathy Fuhrman, Tamara Masiado, Sandra L. Yaich, and Thomas Wasser. "Evaluation and Recommendations from a Study of a Critical-Care Waiting Room." *Journal for Healthcare Quality* 27(4), (2005): 17–25. doi:10.1111/j.1945-1474.2005.tb00564.x
80 Tsai, et al. "Hospital Outpatient Perceptions of the Physical Environment of Waiting Areas."
81 Greaves, Felix, Utz J. Pape, Dominic King, Ara Darzi, Azeem Majeed, Robert M. Wachter, and Christopher Millet. "Associations between Web-Based Patient Ratings and Objective Measures of Hospital Quality." *Archives of Internal Medicine* 172(5), (2012): 435–436. doi:10.1001/archinternmed.2011.1675
82 Luxford, Karen. "Editorial: What Does the Patient Know about Quality?" *International Journal for Quality in Health Care* 24(5), (2012): 439–440. doi:10.1093/inqhc/mzs053
83 Lin, Blossom Yen Ju, Chung Ping Cliff Hsu, Cheng Hua Lee, and Ming Ching Chao. "Patient Satisfaction in Hospital-Based Emergency Departments: Recommendation for Healthcare Management and Policy." *International Journal of Public Policy* 5(2–3), (2010): 175–189. doi:10.1504/IJPP.2010.030602
84 Zeisel, John. *Inquiry by Design: Tools for Environment-Behavior Research.* Monterey, CA: Brooks/Cole Publishing, 1981.
85 Pennachio, "Practice Pointers," (see chap. 2, n. 30).
86 Boyce, John M., and Didier Pittet. "Guideline for Hand Hygiene in Health-care Settings – Recommendations of the Healthcare Infection Control Practices Advisory Committee and the HICPAC/SHEA/APIC/IDSA Hand Hygiene Task Force." *American Journal of Infection Control* 39(8), (2002): S1–S46.
87 Randle, Jacqueline, Mitch Clarke, and Julie Ann Storr. "Hand Hygiene Compliance in Healthcare Workers." *Journal of Hospital Infection* 64, (2006): 205–209. doi:10.1016/j.jhin.2006.06.008
88 Center for Disease Control and Prevention. "Hand Hygiene in Healthcare Settings." Center for Disease Control and Prevention. Accessed August 1, 2013. http://www.cdc.gov/handhygiene/
89 Huisman, E. R. C. M., Ester J. Morales, Joost Van Hoof, and Helianthe S. M. Kort. "Healing Environment: A Review of the Impact of the Physical Environment." *Building and Environment* 58, (2012): 70–80, 74. doi:10.1016/j.buildenv.2012.06.016
90 Tsai, et al., "Hospital Outpatient Perceptions of the Physical Environment of Waiting Areas."
91 Cawthorn, Anne. "A Review of the Literature Surrounding the Research into Aromatherapy." *Complementary Therapies in Nursing & Midwifery* 1(4), (1995): 118–120.
92 Lehrner, Johann, Christine Eckersberger, Peter Walla, G. Pötsch, and L. Deecke. "Ambient Odor of Orange in a Dental Office Reduces Anxiety and Improves Mood in Female Patients." *Physiology & Behavior* 71(1–2), (2000): 83–86. doi:10.1016/S0031-9384(00)00308-5
93 Holm, Lydia, and Laura Fitzmaurice. "Emergency Department Waiting Room Stress: Can Music or Aromatherapy Improve Anxiety Scores?" *Pediatric Emergency Care* 24(12), (2008): 836–838. doi:10.1097/PEC.0b013e31818ea04c
94 Lin, et al., "Patient Satisfaction in Hospital-Based Emergency Departments."
95 Huisman, E. R. C. M. et al., "Healing Environment."
96 Lankford, Mary G., Susan M. Collins, Larry Youngberg, Denise M. Rooney, John Robin Warren, and Gary A. Noskin. "Assessment of Materials Commonly Utilized in Health Care: Implications for

Bacterial Survival and Transmission." *American Journal of Infection Control* 34(5), (2006): 258–263. doi:10.1016/j.ajic.2005.10.008

97 Ulrich, Roger S., Craig Zimring, Xuemei Zhu, Jennifer DuBose, Hyun-Bo Seo, Young-Seon Choi, Xiaobo Quan, and Anjali Joseph. "A Review of the Research Literature on Evidence-Based Healthcare Design." *Health Environments Research & Design Journal* 1(3), (2008): 61–125.

98 Ulrich *et al.*, "A Review of the Research Literature," 13.

99 Quan, Xiaobo, Anjali Joseph, and Matthew Jelen. "Green Cleaning in Healthcare: Current Practices and Questions for Future Research." The Center for Health Design, September, 2011. http://www.healthdesign.org/chd/research/green-cleaning-healthcare-current-practices-and-questions-future-research

100 Green Seal. Accessed August 1, 2013. http://www.greenseal.org/AboutGreenSeal.aspx

101 HermanMiller Healthcare. "Healthier Planet, Healthier People: Hospitals Go Green to 'First Do No Harm.'" HermanMiller Healthcare, 2009. http://www.hermanmiller.com/content/dam/hermanmiller/documents/research_summaries/wp_GreenHospitals.pdf

102 Ananth, Sita, "Building Healing Spaces," *Explore: The Journal of Science and Healing* 4(6), (2008), 393.

103 CDC. *Costs of Falls Among Older Adults*. CDC. Accessed August 1, 2013. http://www.cdc.gov/HomeandRecreationalSafety/Falls/fallcost.html

104 Bergen, Gwendolyn, Li-Hui Chen, Margaret Warner, and Lois A. Fingerhut. *Injury in the United States: 2007 Chartbook*. Hyattsville, MD: National Center for Health Statistics, 2007. See esp. Figure 22–2. http://www.cdc.gov/nchs/data/misc/injury2007.pdf

105 Gulwadi, Gowri Betrabet, and Amy Beth Keller. "Falls in Healthcare Settings." *Healthcare Design*, June 30, 2009. http://www.healthcaredesignmagazine.com/article/falls-healthcare-settings?page=2

106 Goodwin, M. B., and Johanna Irene Westbrook. "An Analysis of Patient Accidents in Hospital." *Australian Clinical Review* 13(3), (1993): 131–149.

107 Gulwadi, Gowri Betrabet, and Margaret P. Calkins. "The Impact of Healthcare Environmental Design on Patient Falls." The Center for Health Design, 2008. http://www.healthdesign.org/sites/default/files/impact_of_healthcare_environment_design_on_patient_falls.pdf

108 Gulwadi and Calkins, "The Impact of Healthcare," 2.

109 Lowes, Robert. "Spot the Safety Hazards in This Office – and Yours." *Medical Economics*, May 7, 2001. http://www.modernmedicine.com/modernmedicine/article/articleDetail.jsp?id=118088

110 Sadler, Blair L., Anjali Joseph, Amy Keller, and Bill Rostenberg. "Using Evidence-Based Environmental Design to Enhance Safety and Quality." IHI Innovation Series White Paper. Cambridge, Massachusetts: Institute for Healthcare Improvement, 2009. http://www.ihi.org/knowledge/Pages/IHIWhitePapers/UsingEvidenceBasedEnvironmentalDesignWhitePaper.aspx

111 Huisman, E. R. C. M. *et al.*, "Healing Environment."

112 OfficeWorks™. "HIPAA Compliance, Work Place Safety, and Universal Precautions," OfficeWorks™, 4, 8. Accessed August 1, 2013. http://www.officeworksrx.com/documents/HIPAAUniversalPrecautionsSafety.pdf

113 Ananth, "Building Healing Spaces," 393.

114 Lowes, "Spot the Safety Hazards in This Office."

115 ECRI Institute. "Are High Risks Putting Your Physician Practices in Jeopardy?" ECRI Institute. Accessed August 1, 2013. https://www.ecri.org/physicianpractice

116 Herczeg, "It's Not Just About Time, (see chap. 2, n. 20).

117 Lerner, Jonathan. "Would You Like a Latte with That Library Card?" *Miller-McCune*, (March–April, 2010): 24–27, 29.

118 Reisman, Anna. "House of Death." The Opinion Pages. *New York Times*, June 2, 2013.

Image Credits

1.03 Plate credit: Dennis O'Brien, Maps and Wayfinding, LLC

1.05 Photo credit (bottom): Aaron Usher III Photography

1.08 Photo credit: Dennis O'Brien, Maps and Wayfinding, LLC

1.14 Photo credit (left and right): The S/L/A/M Collaborative

2.02 Illustration credit: Dennis O'Brien, Maps and Wayfinding, LLC

2.04 Illustration credit: Dennis O'Brien, Maps and Wayfinding, LLC

2.05 Photo credit: Woodruff/Brown Architectural Photography

2.06 Photo credit: John Giammatteo

2.07 Photo credit: John Giammatteo

2.08 Photo credit: Aaron Usher III Photography

2.09 Photo credit: The S/L/A/M Collaborative

2.11 Photo credit: Woodruff/Brown Architectural Photography

2.16 Photo credit: John Giammatteo

2.18 Photo credit: John Giammatteo

2.20 Photo credit: The S/L/A/M Collaborative

2.22 Photo credit: Northern Westchester Hospital

2.24 Photo credit: Woodruff/Brown Architectural Photography

2.25 Photo credit: Woodruff/Brown Architectural Photography

2.30 Photo credit: John Giammatteo

2.31 Photo credit: John Giammatteo

2.35 Photo credit (right): Maggie Dillon, IDeA

2.36 Photo credit: John Giammatteo

3.01 Photo credit: John Giammatteo

3.03 Photo credit: John Giammatteo

3.04 Photo credit: John Giammatteo

3.06 Illustration credit: Sheila F. Cahnman, AIA, ACHA, former Group Vice President, HOK. Credit: Reprinted from *Health Facilities Management* by permission, June 2011, Copyright 2011, by Health Forum, Inc.

3.08 Photo credit: Aaron Usher III Photography

3.10 Photo credit: Aaron Usher III Photography

3.11 Photo credit: Woodruff/Brown Architectural Photography

3.12 Photo credit: The S/L/A/M Collaborative

3.13 Photo credit: Aaron Usher III Photography

3.15 Photo credit: John Giammatteo

4.01 Photo credit: John Giammatteo

4.05 Photo credit: John Giammatteo

4.06 Photo credit: Dawn A. Gum, AIA and IIDA

4.07 Photo credit: Woodruff/Brown Architectural Photography

4.09 Photo credit: John Giammatteo

4.13 Photo credit: John Giammatteo

Index

A

access
   to amenities 3, 123
   to nature 33, 114
   to technology 5, 16, 82
accessibility and ADA guidelines 6, 28, 34, 51, 106, 128
Acoustic Environment Technical Brief
   Green Guide for Health Care™ 88, 102
acoustics *see* noise control
administrative functions 41, 64, 87, 92, 114
advice manuals for physicians 1, 100
Affordable Care Act (ACA) 5
Agency for Research Healthcare and Quality 129
air changes per hour (ACH) 125
air quality 105, 125–6
Albright's *Office Practitioner* 14, 99, 100
alphanumeric information 25, 47; *see also* wayfinding, role in
Altman, Irwin 10, 11, 53
ambient environment *see* Chapter 4
ambulatory care centers 11
American Academy of Healthcare Interior Designers 64
American Art Resources 110, 117, 130
American Hospital Association 38
American Institute of Architects (AIA) 125
   2006 Guidelines for the Design and Construction of Healthcare Facilities 3
American Society of Health, Refrigerating, and Air Conditioning Engineers (ASHRAE) 125
Americans with Disabilities Act (ADA) 6, 28, 34, 51, 106, 128
antimicrobial-resistant bacteria 126
anxiety and medical consultation 39–40, 77
   and privacy 72, 87
   and violations of personal space 11
   and wayfinding 16, 37
appearance
   non-institutional 63
   of office 1, 13, 99
   of physician 1
aquarium, as positive distraction 110, 129

Arneill, Allison 75
Arneill, Bruce and Frasca-Beaulieu, Kerrie 25, 92, 108
aromatherapy 3, 126
arrival 13, 42, 51
art 34, 40, 48, 66, 75, 81, 92, 95, 99, 110, 112
   content guidelines for use in therapeutic settings 115, 117–18
   microaggressions, visual 118
Art Research Institute 110, 117
artificial light *see* lighting
atrium
   Bronson Methodist Hospital 4, 5
   Yale New Haven Hospital 115
attention restoration *see* nature
auditory privacy 87–89
   design considerations 51, 66, 73
   and sound-absorbing carpet 88

B

balanced-budget amendment 3
Barczak, Timothy, office of xiii, 66, 68, 102
bariatric seating 56, 57; *see also* waiting room furniture
Barnes, Marni 33, 34, 37, 38
basic research *see* research design
Bathroom, The 72, 75
BBH Design xiii, 112
Becker, Franklin 75
Benya, James R. 93, 102
Berger, Craig 38
beverage center 123–24
Bodine, Kerry 82, 83
books, role in office of early practitioners 101, 120
borrowed view 30, 111
Bradt, Joke 122
Brady Bunch, The 82
braille and wayfinding 49
brand identity of hospitals 4
Bronson Methodist Hospital 4
Brownsville, Ohio 14
business, of medicine xi, 2

C

cabinets, screening in 101
  storage in 79, 101, 120
café 64, 112, 113, 123; see also beverage center
Cahnman, Sheila xiii, 81, 102
Calori, Chris 38
carpeting
  antimicrobial 126
  cleanliness of 126
  and soft architecture 58, 107
  and sound control 88
Carpman, Janet Reizenstein 34, 36, 38
Carr, Robert 2
Casciato, Daniel 102
case study 9; see also research design
Cathell, Daniel Webster 1, 14, 15, 23, 99, 119
causality 6–8, 9, 63; see also research design
ceiling window as art 113
ceilings
  and acoustics 69, 87, 88
  and height 112
cell phone use 89
Center for Health Design (CHD) 3–4
  and evidence-based design 63
  issue paper on green cleaning 127
  issue paper on sound control 87
  Pebble Project 4
Centers for Disease Control (CDC) 125, 130
cerebral cortex and visual system 106
chairs
  arms as boundaries 55, 56
  bariatric 56, 57
  doctor's waiting room effect 57
  number in waiting room 59
check in and check out 6, 13, 18, 41, 42, 44, 45, 46, 50, 51–2; see also reception area
check in kiosks 51
  Connected Technology Solutions 51
  Patient Passport Express 51
children's area in waiting room 129
choice 10–11, 15, 53, 54, 56, 59, 64, 69, 81, 86, 90, 98, 129, 130; see also control
  in garden 33, 34, 36
choice points for wayfinding 19, 24; see also wayfinding
Church, Thomas 13
Cincinnati Children's Hospital 110
Clarksburg, West Virginia 14, 100
cleanliness 74, 88
  and carpeting 126
  and green issues 127
  and odor 125, 126; see also safety
clinical outcomes and design 2, 3, 4, 7, 8, 9, 11, 31, 33, 34, 40, 54, 59, 89, 95, 112, 127
clutter 17, 21, 86, 95, 96, 101; see also safety
Coastal Connecticut Dentistry 56, 127
Coastal Dermatology 29, 30
Cognition and Environment: Functioning in an Uncertain World 10
cognitive map 16–17
color
  aesthetic considerations 34, 40, 75, 78, 79, 85, 118
  for lighting 75, 93, 95
  for wayfinding 24, 25, 47–8; see also wayfinding
comfort garden, San Francisco General Hospital 35; see also garden
community health centers xi, 85
competence motivation 10, 40, 130
  and Freud, Sigmund 10
  and White, Robert 10
complimentary food and beverages 123; see also beverage center
computer
  for check in 51
  impact on doctor-patient communications (DPC) 82, 84, 90–1
  location of monitor and HIPAA considerations 51–2, 88
  privacy screen for 51
  in waiting room 6, 59, 110; see also electronic medical records, EMRs
conference room, decibel level in 88
Connected Technology Solutions 51
consultation space
  auditory privacy in 87
  and exam space 83
  illumination in 91–2
  Jack-and-Jill model 82–3
  models of 77–83
  temperature in 83, 126
Continuous Ambient Relaxation Environment (C.A.R.E.) Channel 109, 122–3
control
  design considerations for 26, 28, 30, 39, 53, 54, 59, 66, 69, 73, 86, 98, 105
  impact on patients 106, 119
  of infection 86
  of lighting 62, 91, 93, 95
  of music 123
  of noise 88

Index

of signage 17–18, 21, 33
of television 107–9
theme of 10–11, 130
in waiting room 59, 60
control group *see* research design
Cooper, Randy 38
Cooper Marcus, Clare 33, 34, 37, 38
Cornell research on waiting rooms 40, 58
correlation 6, 7–9; *see also* research design
corridor
    storage 71, 87
    and vital signs niche 84
    wayfinding cues in 47, 50, 106
critical care unit, recommendations from 69
Crossing the Quality Chasm 5
cues
    alphanumeric 47
    color, caution in use of 47
    manifest vs. latent 47
    redundant 49
    sensory modality of 49
    view as 50
    for wayfinding 44, 45, 46, 47; *see also* wayfinding
culture
    consumer 2
    of correctional facilities 69
    of medicine 16, 85

D

Danbury Hospital Pulmonary Department 41
decision points *see* wayfinding
defensible space theory 42–3
    and Newman, Oscar 42
degree of statistical significance *see* research design
dependent variable 6, 7; *see also* experiment; *see also* research design
Design that Cares: Planning Health Facilities for Patients and Visitors 38
Devlin, Ann Sloan i, 75, 103
Dietrick, Lynn 123
Dileo, Cheryl 122
directional signs *see* signs, types
disposal of waste 36, 70, 71, 86; *see also* waste
distractions *see* positive distractions
docs-in-a-box 16
doctor-patient communication 89–91
Doctor Peter Centre, Vancouver 32, 33
doctor's waiting room effect 57
Dollars to Doctors or Diplomacy and Prosperity in Medical Practice 14, 120

doors and screening 65, 66, 67, 88, 101, 102, 120, 121
dosage of analgesics and design 2, 31, 110
dynamic lighting *see* lighting

E

effect size 8
egress
    and lighting 93
    and safety 129
    and saving face 97
EKG cart, location of 43, 81
electrical outlets
    in furniture 59
    standard location of 83
electronic medical records (EMRs)
    design of location for 83–4
    and doctor patient communication 89–91
    and HIPAA 87
    requirement to use 5
Emergency Care Research Institute (ECRI) 129
employees *see* staff
entrance
    and parking 18, 25, 27, 28, 29
    porte-cochère 25, 26
    welcoming 117
Environmental Design Research Association (edra) xiii, 82
Europe
    aromatherapy use in 126
    exam room layout in 81
evaluation
    HCAHPS xi
    of medicine 39
    patient satisfaction 125
    post occupancy 9
event schema 13; *see also* script
evidence-based design
    and furnishings 63
    and Ripple Database 4
    role of xi, 2–3
evolutionary
    human characteristics and cognition 9–10, 56
    response to nature 115
exam room
    auditory privacy in 87–8
    cabinetry 79, 80
    clinical vs. family zones of use 81
    clutter 86
    combined with consultation space 77
    design considerations 78, 115

dressing and undressing, considerations for 85–6
functional aspects of 74, 78, 79, 80, 81, 85, 86, 125
historical examples of 99–101
hotelling 84
infection control in 86
layouts 81, 82
lighting in 92
location options 83
orientation of exam table 82–3
monitor position and EMRs in 90–1
patient privacy in 85–6
screening in 78–9
sharps and waste disposal in 86–7
sinks 84
size of 78
standardization 83
storage in 83, 84
temperature in 126
time spent in 40, 53
experiment
between subjects 6
dependent variable 6, 7
field 107
independent variable 6, 7
true 6, 9; *see also* research design
expert, definition of 6

F

fabrics
manufacturers 64
non-institutional appearance 63, 64
selection criteria 64
falls and design-related issues 83, 128–9
family
resource center 120, 121
seating for 56, 81, 83, 159
familiarity and wayfinding 47
fences as thematic and wayfinding elements 37
Fischer, Joey 112, 117
Art Research Institute Limited 110, 117
and Stanford 117
Fitzmaurice, Laura 126
Flexibility of technology 90, 93
flooring
carpeting 126
green considerations 127–8
and safety 128
as wayfinding aids 47, 48
Florence, Italy
Meyer Children's Hospital and transparency 50

fluorescent lighting
considerations 92, 93, 112
vs. full spectrum 63
vs. incandescent 62; *see also* lighting
Flynn, John E. 92, 102
Follis, John 38
food *see* beverage center
formaldehyde in materials 63
Fort Belvoir Community Hospital design 5
Frampton, Susan 102
Freud, Sigmund 10
front vs. back of house metaphor 40, 41, 42, 43, 64
Fulefor design group 129; *see also* waiting room
furniture
bariatric 56, 57
in children's area 129
in exam room 81, 82
influence of hospitality movement on 63, 64
magazine/brochure rack 60, 120, 121
number of seats 54–5, 59
seating clusters 53, 54, 47, 60, 64, 110
shelving 70, 121
in staff lounge 69–70
in waiting area 11, 39, 40, 53–61, 110
further reading 38, 75, 102, 130

G

Gaerig, Chris 130
garden
access for staff 114
desirable and undesirable qualities in 34
furnishings in 34–6
healing 33
labyrinth 113
lighting in 38
San Francisco General Hospital comfort garden 35
seasonal plantings in 31
seating in 34–36
theory of supportive gardens 33
trash receptacles 34, 36
water elements in 114
wayfinding elements in 36–7
Gesler, Wilbert M. 38
Giammatteo, John xiii, 45, 53, 55, 67, 73, 78, 79, 80, 101, 107, 111, 121, 149, 150
Gilpin, Laura 115, 118, 131
Gosling, Samuel 1, 96
Snoop: What Your Stuff Says About You 1–2
GPS and wayfinding 16

Index 155

graphic designers and wayfinding 16, 17, 24, 38, 49
green cleaning 127, 128
   and asthma 127
   and dermatitis 127
   floor materials 128
   Green Guide for Health Care™ 88
   Green Seal cleaners 128, 130
   and housekeeping closet 127
   and pregnancy 127
green design and sustainability 5
Green Seal 128, 130
Griffin Hospital, Derby, Connecticut xiii, 26, 29, 32, 52, 57, 92–3, 113, 120, 121
   parking in 26, 27
   Planetree model 26
group practice
   signage for 23
   space use in 66–7, 83–5
group workspace and medical culture 85
Guidelines for the Design and Construction of Health Care Facilities (AIA, 2006) 3
Gulwadi, Gowri Betrabet 102, 128
Gum, Dawn A. xiii, 111, 112, 150

H
Hall, Edward T. 55
Hamilton, D. Kirk 69, 75
handicap access
   Americans with Disabilities Act (ADA) 6
   parking 25, 28
   reception desk 51
   toilet room 59
   and universal design, 28, 128
   waiting room 59
Harkness, Sarah P. 38
Hasbro Children's Hospital, Providence, Rhode Island 35, 37, 110
Hathorn, Kathy 118, 130
hazardous waste, disposal and storage of 81, 86; *see also* waste
headphones
   hygiene 108, 122
   and music 122, 123
headwall in same-handed and mirror image rooms 83
healing garden 5, 33, 34; *see also* garden
Healing Gardens: Therapeutic Benefits and Design Recommendations 33, 38
Healing HealthCare Systems® 110, 122, 123
Health Care without Harm 128

Health Facilities Management magazine xiii, 81, 150
Health Insurance Portability and Accountability Act (HIPAA)
   design considerations for 6, 51, 69, 87, 88, 97, 129
health outcomes
   and light 95
   and nature 30
   and positive distractions 59
   and sense of control 54, 59
   and supportive garden theory 33
   and toxins 127
health and safety regulations 36, 44, 88, 128, 129
Healthcare Design Conference 58, 59, 60, 63
Healthcare Design Magazine 118
Healthier Hospitals Initiative (HHI)
   White paper on green cleaning 127
heating, ventilation, and air conditioning (HVAC)
   air changes per hour (ACH) 125
   odor control 125, 126
   ventilation 125, 127
Herczeg, Laszlo 75
Herman Miller
   Healthier Planet, Healthier People 128
   Herman Miller Healthcare 88
   Nemschoff 64
Herzog, Thomas 115
Hidden Dimension, The 55
hierarchical organization of space 40, 41, 42, 87, 98
hierarchy of medicine 85
Hilton, B. Ann 88
Hippocrates and Planetree 3
historical perspective on medicine i, xi, 1, 11, 13, 14, 15, 23, 99, 100, 119, 120
Holm, Lydia 126
hospice unit, schema of 130
hospital acquired infection (HAI) 8, 127
Hospital Consumer Assessment of Healthcare Providers and Systems (HCAHPS) xi
Hospital da Luz, Lisbon, Portugal 113
Hospital for a Healthy Environment (H2E) 5; *see also* Practice Greenhealth
hotelling and exam room use 84
How to Succeed in the Practice of Medicine 14
Huisman, E. R. C. M. 129, 130
humans
   as limited information processors 13, 14
   and mastery 10, 59
   as model makers 10

preference for prospect and refuge 56, 106
  as territorial 10, 11
Humanscape: Environments for People 10
hygiene articles of early practitioners 87, 101

I

IDeA xiii, 72, 112, 150
Idealized Design of Clinical Offices Practices (IDCOP) 5
identification in wayfinding 19, 23; see also wayfinding
identity, clues to 1–2, 4, 13, 14, 15, 18, 19, 23, 24, 37
illumination see lighting
image of medical facilities
  hospital as hotel 5, 25, 64, 72
  hospitality 63
impression formation
  of medical facilities 1–2
  of physicians 1–2; see also schema
incandescent lighting see lighting
independent variable 6, 7; see also experiment; see also research design
infection
  control 8, 86, 87, 88, 117, 125
  rates of 2, 4, 8
information
  alphanumeric 24, 47
  overload 23, 118; see also wayfinding
Institute for Healthcare Improvement (IHI) 5, 129
Institute of Medicine (IOM) 5
Interior Architecture & Design, PLLC xiii, 111
interior finishes see carpeting; see walls
Internet
  patient use of 5, 16, 59, 82, 95, 130
  server room 5, 90
  technology for 57, 58, 59, 64, 98, 106, 110

J

Joseph, Anjali 102, 103, 131

K

Kaiser Permanente Medical Center 129
Kaplan, Rachel 10, 30, 31
Kaplan, Stephen 10, 30, 31
Keep It Simple Stupid (KISS) Principle 23
Kira, Alexander 72, 75
Kohli, Neeraj, office of xiii, 52, 70, 71, 72, 80, 96, 109, 116, 117, 124

L

laboratory
  location 43, 68–9
  specimen processing 74
labyrinth
  California Pacific Medical Center 113
  restorative effect of 113; see also garden
landmarks, as wayfinding aids see wayfinding
landscaping
  borrowed landscapes in 30; see also borrowed landscapes
  desirable and undesirable qualities in 31–4
  entrance 13, 25, 28, 29, 37
  exterior 28–38
  lighting 38
  outdoor furnishings 34–5, 36
  parking 26–7
  seasonal foliage in 31
  water elements in 30, 31, 32, 33
  wayfinding elements in 36–7
Langer, Ellen 54
Las Vegas syndrome 17
laundry, soiled linen 70, 101
layout see exam room layout; see spatial continuum
learned helplessness theory 77
  and Maier, Steven 10
  and Seligman, Martin 10
Leather, Phil 75
Leemis, Caroline 110, 123, 131
legibility 17, 49; see also wayfinding
lettering on signs 19, 23
Lidwell, William 38
lighting
  characteristics, 62, 93, 95,
  clerestory 94, 111
  control of glare 62, 75, 93, 112
  effects on staff 92, 95
  in examination room 83, 91, 92
  and fatigue 95
  garden 38
  natural 93–4
  personal control 62, 95
  skylights 95
  sunlight 34, 62, 63, 92, 112
  task 60, 61, 62, 95
  types of 62, 63, 91, 92, 93, 95, 112
  in waiting room 62
limited processing capacity of humans 9, 13, 14
Lisbon, Portugal 32, 34, 36, 113
Lisbon University Institute 21, 24, 26, 113
location of medical facilities
  community v. hospital based 15–16
  historical perspective 115
  implications for medical office 115

Index

implications for wayfinding 16–17
  medical mall 16
lockers, staff 70
lounge, staff 69–70, 73
Lucile Packard Children's Hospital 53
Lynch, Kevin 16, 26

M

magazines
  availability 59, 100, 107, 109, 120
  racks and shelving 60, 121
  selection of 119, 120
Maier, Steven 10
Malkin, Jain 59, 64, 69, 70, 72, 74, 75, 89
managed care 14
Manning, Harley 82, 83
maps, GPS 16
Marietta, Ohio 100
massage
  and aromatherapy 126
  in Planetree hospitals 3
Mathews, Joseph McDowell 14, 23, 100
Maxwell, John C. 39
Mayo Clinic
  Center for Innovation 82
  collaboration with Steelcase 64, 82
  Jack-and-Jill model 82–3
  research tradition 82
  See, Plan, Act, Refine, Communicate (SPARC) innovation program 64
Mazer, Susan E. 108, 109, 122, 131
McColl, Shelley L. 103
medical chart racks, padding for 88
medical displays
  of early practitioners 119–120
  effect on patients 119
medical mall
  connotation of 16
  docs-in-a-box 16
medical records, electronic (EMRs) *see* electronic medical records (EMRs)
Medicare reimbursement 3–4, 89
Medicine Moves to the Mall 16
mental representation *see* schema
mercury waste 5
meta-analysis 6, 8, 9, 122
Methicillin-resistant Staphylococcus aureus (MRSA) 125
Meyer Children's Hospital, Florence, Italy 50
microaggression, visual 118
Microsoft templates for office planning 84

millennials and multi-tasking 13–14
Miller, George, and specification of memory information limit 13
mobility challenges 28, 51, 62, 128
models of consultation 77
  exam room layouts 81–2
  "having a seat at the table" 82
  Jack-and-Jill layout 82–3
  location of consultation and exam spaces 83
  same-handed vs. mirror-image rooms 83
  shared functions 84–5
  traditional exam room layout 78–81
Mollerup, Per 38
multi-method strategies for research 8–9
multi-tasking, and performance 14, 90
music
  C.A.R.E. channel 109, 122
  genres 122
  guidelines for selection 122, 123
  headphones and hygiene 108, 122
  headphones for patients 172
  Healing HealthCare Systems® 110, 122, 123
  and health outcomes 122
  Music Care® 123
  patient-provided 123

N

Nasar, Jack L. 103
National Health Service, United Kingdom 125
National Institute of Building Science 2
natural light, effects of 62, 63, 93–4, 95, 100, 110, 112,
nature/natural elements
  attention restoration 30, 31
  ceiling and wall murals 112, 113
  as healing garden 33
  impact of 30, 31
  and Kaplan, Rachel and Stephen 30, 31
  plants 34, 99, 105, 114, 116–17
  preferred elements in 31
  substitutes for 117
  and Ulrich, Roger S. 31, 33, 34, 75, 103, 130, 111, 115, 118, 131
  view to 30, 110
  water elements in 31, 32, 33
near patient alcohol hand rubs (NPAHs) 125
Nemschoff 64; *see also* Herman Miller
Newhill, Christina E. 98
Newman, Oscar 42
Nightingale award 58
noise

Acoustic Environment Technical Brief 88
cell phone policy 89
decibel levels 87
and privacy 87
sound-proofing 69, 72, 87, 88
sources 87, 88
speech privacy 87–8; *see also* music
Northern Westchester Hospital xiii, 58, 73, 149
nosocomial infection *see* hospital acquired infection (HAI)
nurse preparation area 64–6
nurse station 64–7; *see also* vital signs station

O

O'Brien, Dennis xiii, 20, 26, 41, 43, 47, 149
occupational hazards and safety regulations 129; *see also* waste
Occupational Safety and Health Administration (OSHA) 36, 128
odor control 125, 126; *see also* ventilation
office displays
   of early practitioners 100, 101, 119–20
   today 40, 75, 95, 96, 99, 110, 114, 116, 118, 119
office exterior 15, 16, 23, 28, 42, 92, 129
office location *see* location of medical facilities
office personalization 58, 95
   for physician 95–6
   for psychotherapist 99
   for staff 95
Office Works™ 119, 131
180-degree principle 106–7
orientation
   aids 37, 50, 106; *see also* wayfinding
   of patient exam table 78, 81
Outside In: The Power of Putting Customers at the Center of Your Business 82
overload *see* information

P

p value 8, 9; *see also* probability value
pain control reduction
   through lighting 63
   through music 120, 122, 123
   through nature 11, 110
parking 25–8
   and ADA 28
   clustering and number
   and front entrance 25, 26, 29
   and landscaping 27, 29
   music in 26

necessary vs. sufficient 28
planning for 26
seating in 26, 27
signage 25, 26, 29
universal design 28
patient
   anxiety 11, 16, 37, 39, 40, 72, 77, 87, 98, 110, 122, 126, 130
   communication about 69; *see also* physician/patient communication
   communication with 3, 59, 82, 83, 89–91, 97
   consumerism xi, 2, 3, 4, 130
   education 106
   flow 40–1, 42, 43, 44, 69, 97
   information retention 77
   perception of healthcare environment 1, 59, 109
   in Planetree model 3, 4, 25, 26, 105, 108, 123, 130
   resource center 121
   safety 15, 28, 36, 44, 93, 128–30;
Patient Passport Express 51
patient personal health information (PHI) 129
patient privacy
   auditory 51, 87–8
   in exam space 66–7. 81–2, 111
   in garden 33
   in hallways 42
   and HIPAA 51–2, 69
   historically 87, 100
   in psychotherapy 97–8
   in restroom 72, 83, 74
   and state of undress 85–6
   in waiting room 53–4, 55, 64
The Patient Protection and Affordable Care Act (PPACA) or (ACA) 5
   Medicare reimbursement 5, 89
patient resource center, in Planetree model 120, 121
patient-centered care 29, 80, 89, 90, 92
   movement 3–4
Pearson product-moment correlation (Pearson's *r*) 7, 9
Pebble Project, The 4, 127
   Ripple database 4
personal space
   bubble 55
   definition 55
   and territoriality 10
   in waiting room 53, 55–6
personalization
   importance of diplomas and credentials 1, 95, 96, 99

Index

159

in office suite 58, 95–6
status for psychotherapist and identity 99
pharmacy location 43, 44
phlebotomy 66, 67
photographs
and personalization 99
as substitute for nature 105, 109, 111, 117
physical traces
design implications 125
and John Zeisel 125, 131
physician
clues to expertise 1–2
identity 1
schema 1, 2 13
shortage 39
physician appearance
early 20th century 1
schema 1, 2, 13
white coat effect 13
Physician Himself and What He Should Add to His Scientific Acquirements, The 1, 14
physician's practice, the
appearance from the street 14, 15, 20, 21, 25
historical perspectives 1, 14–15, 23, 99–101, 119, 120
physician-patient communication
consultation room and 82–3
EMRs 89–91
telemedicine and teletherapy 97–8
waiting time 53
physiological indicators of stress and design 39, 107–8, 116, 122
piano, in Planetree model 3, 5
pictograms
ambiguous 25; *see also* wayfinding
universal 25
Planetree
design elements 25, 26, 105, 108, 123
model of patient-centered care 3
origins and mission 3
role of senses in 3, 123
Thieriot, Angelica 3
planning considerations
outdoor spaces 34, 37
parking/traffic 26–8
for seating 59
spatial layout 40–2
technology 90
plants, live *see* nature, plants
plumbing chase
and mirror-image rooms, same-handed rooms 83

Pollet, Dorothy 38
porte cochère, at entrance 25, 26
positive distractions
aquariums as 92, 110
and aromatherapy 3, 126
art and 3, 34, 39, 40, 52, 66, 75, 92, 95, 99, 117–18
in exam room 79, 81, 116
music as 120–3
nature as 109–10, 113, 114, 116
pain reduction in 110
plants as 116–17
self-paced 120, 121
television as 107–9; *see also* television
view as 97, 110, 111–12, 113
water as 114–16
post occupancy evaluation (POE) 6, 9
Practice Greenhealth 5
pre-post design *see* research design
predictability *see* schema
Press Ganey patient satisfaction survey 2, 53
primary care physician shortage 2
privacy *see* patient privacy
privacy screen for computer 51
private vs. semi-private rooms 3, 4, 5
probability value 8; *see also* significance level
proxemics 55
and E. T. Hall 55
zones: intimate, personal, social, public 55
Pruyn, Ad 108
psychotherapy office
décor 99
diplomas and credentials 99
restrooms and location 98
security issues 98–9
spatial layout 97
teletherapy 97–8
view 97
public, semi-public, semi-private, and private space 42, 43, 98

R

racks
brochure 71
magazine 60
for medical implements 79, 80, 83
ramps and handicapped accessibility 6, 28, 29
random assignment to condition *see* research design
rates of infection 2, 4, 8, 125
reading material

availability of 60, 61, 75, 92, 109, 120, 121
  content of 119, 120
  as self-paced distraction 120
real estate costs 15
reception area
  as bookends of visit 42, 50, 51
  check in stations 42, 45, 46
  HIPAA considerations 51–2
  kiosks 51
  Patient Passport Express 51
  transaction counter and shape 51
  window position (open vs. closed) 51
  wheelchair accommodation 51
Regard™ line for Nurture® by Steelcase 58, 59
regression 7; see also research design
regulations
  HIPAA 6, 51, 69, 87, 88, 97, 129
  OSHA 36
  parking 28
  safety 128, 129
Reis, Shmuel 89, 90, 103
research design
  case study 9
  causality 6–8, 9
  control group 8, 9, 122
  correlation 7, 8, 9
  dependent variable 6, 7
  difficulty in healthcare environments 9
  effect size 8
  independent variable 6, 7
  meta-analysis 8, 9, 122
  objective data 3, 8
  POE 9
  practical significance 8
  pre-post design 9
  probability value 8
  random assignment to condition 6, 7, 9, 82
  sample size 8
  self-report data 2, 3
  statistical significance 6, 8, 9
  subjective data 2, 3
  true experiment 6, 9
restroom
  acoustical privacy in 72
  anxiety about use of 72
  appearance of 71, 72
  ceramic tile 71, 72, 75, 128
  cleanliness and maintenance in 72, 74–75
  gender neutral 74
  handicapped access 6
  lighting in 75

location 42, 50, 73
  number of 74
  paper towels vs. hand dryer in 75
  for psychotherapy practice 98
  specimen pass-through 74
  staff 69, 73
  storage in 74
  waste disposal in 75
Robbins, Saul 99
Rodin, Judith 54

S
safety
  by association 128
  and carpeting 126, 128
  checklist 129
  by design 128–9
  exterior 129
  falls 128, 129
  interior 129–30
  and storage 129
satisfaction measure, Hospital Consumer Assessment of Healthcare Providers and Systems (HCAHPS) xi
scaffolding functions
  laboratory 68, 69
  nurse station 65
  staff preparation 65
  storage 65
  traffic flow 41, 43, 64, 66
  vital signs 65, 66, 67
schema
  expectations of medical care 84, 105, 106, 128, 130
  expectations of spatial organization 16, 43
  humans as model makers 10
  of permission 106
  of physician and office 1, 13, 14, 15, 16, 50, 96, 130; see also script
screening
  by early practitioners 87
  of equipment 65, 67, 69, 101, 102, 112
  of medical waste 86
  for privacy 66, 78, 79, 85
script
  event schema 13; see also schema
  for physician visit 50
seating
  bariatric 56, 57
  calculating number needed 59
  choice of 53, 54, 55, 56, 59

Index

for staff lounge 69, 70
types of 56, 64
upholstery fabric 64
in waiting room 53, 54, 55, 56, 57, 58, 60, 61; *see also* furniture
seating arrangement
   personal space and 55, 56, 57
   territoriality and 53, 54, 57
security in psychotherapy offices 97, 98–9
self-congruity theory 2
self-paced distraction 109, 120
Seligman, Martin 10, 77
senses, the
   air quality and odor 125
   aromatherapy 126
   cleanliness and odor 126
   cleanliness and carpeting 126
   green cleaning 127
   role of in Planetree model 3, 25, 105, 108, 123
   temperature and thermal comfort 126
   vision, role of as major sense 106
Shachak, Aviv 89, 90
shade, in office landscape 5, 34
sharps, disposal of 86; *see also* waste, hazardous
shelter
   from elements 34
   porte-cochère 25, 26
Shepley, Mardelle McCuskey 69, 75
shopping, aspirational and medicine 2
sick people's atmosphere 105
sign *see* signage
sign types
   description 19, 20
   destination 18, 19, 47
   directional 19, 20, 21, 25, 72
   identification 19, 20
   overhead 106
   pictogram 25
   prohibition 19
   regulation 19, 20
   warning 19; *see also* wayfinding
signage
   character in community 17–18
   and choice points 19, 24
   clutter 17, 21
   consistency 17
   for daytime vs. nighttime 21, 23
   for group practice 23, 24
   historical reflections 23
   and identity 17–18, 19
   Las Vegas syndrome 17
   legibility 17, 49
   program 17, 18, 49
   as public relations 15
   as redundant cues 49
   types *see* sign types
significance level 6, 8, 9; *see also* probability value
   meaning of .05 8
silent partner, the 100–1
Simpson, Susan 98
single brew coffee machine 69, 123, 124; *see also* beverage center
single occupancy rooms, AIA recommendations for 3
sinks
   centralized vs. decentralized 84
   location in exam room 79, 80, 81
site plan for parking 26
size
   of art 116, 118
   of exam room 78
   of furniture 36, 56, 67, 64
S/L/A/M Collaborative, The xiii, 29, 32, 42, 44, 45, 46, 48, 53, 55, 57, 58, 60, 61, 67, 73, 78, 79, 80, 92, 93, 101, 107, 111, 113, 114, 121, 149, 150
Sloan, Dr. Herbert Elias 23, 100
smells *see* odor control; *see also* ventilation
Smidts, Ale 108
Smilow Cancer Center, New Haven, Connecticut 110, 115
Smith, Dallas 108, 122, 131
Smitshuijzen, Edo 38
social desirability, effects on research validity 3
social support
   design considerations for 59
   in gardens 33
Society for Experiential Graphic Design (SEGD) 49
soft architecture 58, 62
Sommer, Robert 11, 58
Sound Choices: Using Music to design the Environments in Which You Live, Work, and Heal 122, 131
sound control *see* auditory privacy
space *see* spatial continuum
space planning *see* planning considerations
SPARC
   See, Plan, Act, Refine, Communicate innovation program 64
   Steelcase partnership with Mayo Clinic 64, 82; *see also* Mayo Clinic
spatial continuum

and defensible space theory 42–3
in exam room layout 81, 82
hierarchy of public to private 43, 44
spatial zones 41, 42, 43, 69
and Hall, E. T. 55
and proxemics 55
specimen pass through 74
speech privacy 87, 88, 89
plenum and 87
spittoon 100
spotting safety hazards 129; see also safety
staff
administrative vs. clinical spaces 41
design considerations for 114
food 69
lockers 70
lounge 69–70
outdoor space for 30, 38
preparation areas 64
privacy issues 87
restroom 73
statistical significance
explanatory power 9
meaning of 8
vs. practical significance 8–9
Steelcase
healthcare line 64, 82
Regard™ line for Nurture® 58, 59
storage
location 65, 66, 70–1
in restroom 74
safety considerations 74, 129
stress see anxiety; see also positive distractions
stress reduction
and lighting 63, 110–11
and nature 30, 31, 33, 69, 114, 116, 117
and positive distraction 107, 108, 109, 122, 123
and theory of supported design 59, 130
and theory of supportive gardens 33
through signage 47
study of studies see meta-analysis
Sue, Derald Wing, and microaggressions 118
sunlight
in garden 34
and glare 62; see also lighting
and health 63, 112
in waiting room 62, 112
sustainability 5; see also green design
symbols
ambiguous 25

international system of 71; see also signage
symbol systems see wayfinding

T
table lamp 10, 54, 62, 92, 93, 112; see also furniture
adjustment and patient control 10, 54, 59, 60, 62, 91, 92, 93, 95, 106, 112
location 62
touch lamps 62
technology
at check in 51
and doctor-patient communication 89–90
and electronic medical records (EMRs) 88–9, 90
hotelling 84
monitor placement 90, 91
and sustainability 5
in waiting room 57, 58, 59, 110
telemedicine 97–8
telephone
and auditory privacy 88, 89
and noise 88, 89
teletherapy, design considerations for 97–8
television
alternatives to 54, 109–10
debate surrounding 107–8
nature and music loop 109
negative effects of 108
perception of time passage 109
as positive distraction 107, 109
territoriality
and defensible space theory 42–3
and opportunities for control 10
prerogatives for 43
types of (primary, secondary, tertiary) 11
and waiting room seating 11, 53, 54
themes of book xi, 1, 9–10, 13, 15, 33, 36, 84, 93, 130
theory of supported design 59
Thieriot, Angelica, and Planetree 3
Thundermist Health Center 21, 22, 46, 85, 91, 94
toilet room 71; see also restroom
nomenclature 71
traffic pattern
and exterior backtracking 26
and interior progression 42
trash containers
exterior 26, 34, 36
and screening 86, 101
in waiting room 129
and waste 125; see also waste

Index

trees
  positive qualities of 28, 34
  pruning and safety 21, 129
  as shade 5
Trulove, James Grayson 38
types of signs *see* signs, types

U
Uebele, Andreas 38
Ulrich, Roger S. 31, 33, 34, 75, 103, 110, 111, 115, 118, 131
universal design philosophy 28, 128 69
University of Michigan Medical Center 69
upholstery fabric 64
urinalysis, design implications for 68, 74
Usher, Aaron xiii, 22, 46, 85, 91, 94, 149, 150

V
vancomycin-resistant enterococci (VRE) 126
variable *see* research design
Veitch, Jennifer A. 103
ventilation 125, 127
  air changes 125; *see also* odor control
view
  of nature 39, 69, 97, 106, 111, 112, 114, 117, 118
  as wayfinding cue 50
vinyl flooring 126
Vision 3 Architects xiii, 22, 46, 85, 91, 94
visitors
  accommodation for 30, 34, 40, 47, 69, 73, 123
  in exam room 81, 83
visual art *see* positive distractions
visual system, importance of 106
vital signs station
  linear progression of in medical suite 42
  location 66, 67; *see also* nurse station
  niche model 66
  size 66
volatile organic compounds (VOC), health risks of 63

W
waiting room; *see also* reception area
  aquarium in 110, 129
  attractiveness of 40, 58, 112
  average waiting time in 53
  children's area 129
  Cornell research on 40, 58
  doctor's waiting room effect 57
  food in 123, 124
  Fulefor suggestions 129
  furnishings and décor in 60, 61, 63, 64, 92, 121
  lighting in 58, 59, 60, 61, 62, 63, 91, 92, 93, 94, 95, 110
  music in 93, 109, 121, 122, 123
  nature in 105, 109, 110, 111
  noise reduction 126
  patient control in 59, 60, 61, 62
  personal space and territoriality in 11, 53, 54, 55, 56, 57
  plants 105, 116–17, 129
  reading material in 120, 121
  Regard™ line for Nurture® by Steelcase 58, 59
  restroom proximity to 73–4
  seating arrangement in 53, 54, 55, 56, 57
  seating requirements in 59
  technology in 57, 58, 59, 64, 110
  vista in 57, 110, 112;
walls
  and noise reduction 69, 87, 88
  and privacy 69
waste
  hazardous 81, 86
  and infection control 4, 86, 87, 88, 125
water features
  caution using 115
  human preference for 31, 115
  maintenance of 115
  as positive distraction 30, 32, 33, 114, 115, 118
wayfinding
  aids 18, 19, 47
  choice points 19
  color, considerations in use 25, 47–8
  and cognitive mapping 16
  cues 44, 47, 49; *see also* cues
  entrance 25
  floor identification 24, 49
  and GPS navigation systems 16
  Hotel California lyrics 47
  importance of 16, 17
  landmarks in 16, 48, 106
  legibility 17, 49
  in multi-level buildings 24
  in multiple languages 47
  O'Brien, Dennis, Maps and Wayfinding, LLC xiii, 20, 26, 41, 43, 47, 149
  orientation 37, 50, 106
  overload 17, 23, 118
  pictograms 25
  redundant cues 49
  symbol systems 18
  view as cue 50, 106

and visual clutter 17, 21
websites and wayfinding information 17
see also signage; *see also* sign types
Weidman, Ted 103
what and where systems 14
wheelchair access 28, 24, 51, 57, 59, 129; *see also* handicap access
White, Robert, and competency motivation 10
white coat syndrome 13
Whole Building Design Guide 2
wi-fi
   in office suite 59
   in waiting room 6
windows
   clerestory 94, 111
   control of glare 62, 93, 112
   daylight and 93
   in exam room 78
   productivity and 111
   for psychotherapy office 97, 99
   reception 6, 51, 97
   signage displayed in 23
   size of as percentage of window wall 112
   staff and 111
   views to nature and 31
   vista provided by 50
   in waiting room 100, 112
Women and Infants Center for Reproduction and Infertility xiii, 66, 60, 79, 86, 108, 124
Women and Infants Hospital of Rhode Island 24, 65, 84
Wood, Nathan Elliott 14, 120
Woodruff/Brown Architectural Photography 44, 48, 60, 61, 92, 113, 149, 150
workstations
   niche for 43, 81, 84, 85
   in waiting room 64

Y

Yale New Haven Hospital xiii, 37, 53, 54, 108
   atrium 115

Z

Zeisel, John 125, 131